Hospital Preaching as Informed by Bedside Listening

A Homiletical Guide for Preachers, Pastors, and Chaplains in Hospital, Hospice, Prison, and Nursing Home Ministries

Cajetan N. Ihewulezi

UNIVERSITY PRESS OF AMERICA,® INC.
Lanham • Boulder • New York • Toronto • Plymouth, UK

University Press of America,® Inc.
4501 Forbes Boulevard
Suite 200
Lanham, Maryland 20706
UPA Acquisitions Department (301) 459-3366

Estover Road
Plymouth PL6 7PY
United Kingdom

Printed in the United States of America
British Library Cataloging in Publication Information Available

Library of Congress Control Number: 2010931098
ISBN: 978-0-7618-5292-6 (paperback : alk. paper)
eISBN: 978-0-7618-5293-3

∞™ The paper used in this publication meets the minimum requirements of American National Standard for Information Sciences—Permanence of Paper for Printed Library Materials, ANSI/NISO Z39.48-1992.

To all patients in hospice care

Contents

Acknowledgments

I was blessed with certain people without whom I would have found it more difficult to accomplish this research. In Fr. George Boudreau, O.P., I found a wonderful advisor who directed me well. I am grateful.

My thanks also go to my reader, Fr. Charles Hart, OFM. His powerful suggestions opened my eyes to some areas of my ministry. His contributions enriched my research. I was also blessed with a dedicated editor, Kathleen Tehan, who not only gave me the required support but also with her writing skills, helped me to make this work more interesting to read. For all the support and suggestions Ann Garrido gave me, I am thankful.

In providing assistance and support to help me gather valuable information, I am also most appreciative of the staff and patients of Missouri Baptist Medical Center, Barnes Jewish Hospital, St Anthony's Hospital, and Forest Park Hospital. Last but not least, I thank M. Cristina Stevens for reviewing this book.

Introduction

Having been a pastor of a church for many years before working as a hospital chaplain, I have discovered that more intentional hospital bedside listening to the stories and experiences of the sick is very necessary for effective hospital preaching to the hospital community. The patients' stories and experiences are valuable resources that can be utilized in the preparation and delivery of more effective homilies to the hospital community which is made up of the sick, their families, and the hospital staff. Such intentional bedside listening and the preaching that results from listening are important for addressing the problems of the sick.

In most churches, Sunday homilies do not effectively address the problems of the sick. I discovered this problem as a pastor of a large congregation in Nigeria. My four associate pastors and I tried to minister to the sick in the hospitals within the geographical boundaries of our parish, but we did not have enough time to listen to their stories. On coming to America, I found evidence of the same problem. After serving in a parish and working among the sick here in the United States for the past six years, I also discovered that most Sunday homilies address the moral, social, economic, and political problems of the healthy members of the churches. They do not however, speak so directly to the sick.

There is great need to sit down face to face and attentively listen to the stories, experiences, and feelings of the sick. Bedside encounters with patients can inform the preacher (chaplain or pastoral minister) and can result in more effective liturgical preaching in hospital, hospice, and nursing home settings. Through the interaction of patients' stories with biblical texts, this preaching may contribute to, complement, and enhance the emotional, spiritual, and physical healing of the patient as well as the community. The sick, along with their families and friends, need the Sunday sermons and if possible daily liturgical homilies that address specific problems related to illness, such as: pain, guilt, shame, punishment, re-definition, anger, depression, sadness, regression, isolation, abandonment, habit, addiction, grief, and loss.

Because illness most often separates the sick from their communities, the sick need the type of hospitality that would provide them the opportunity to express themselves. If the sick hear their stories or stories similar to their own being shared with the liturgical community, they may feel more a part of their community while the people of their community, in turn, better understand the contributions of the sick. The feelings, responses, and attitudes that surround the stories of the sick can act as effective means of proclaiming the gospel to the community as well as to other patients.

This project is aimed at improving the pastoral care ministry of the sick. This pastoral approach will provide a homiletical guide for preachers, pastors, and chaplains involved in hospital, hospice, and nursing home ministries. It will also help pastoral ministers to develop better skills of listening to the stories and experiences of the sick as well as the ability to use these stories and experiences in the proclamation of the gospel. This approach may assist them in preparing more effective homilies to address the concerns of the sick. When a pastoral minister provides opportunities for the sick to tell their stories and listens attentively to them, patients feel that someone cares about their pain and sorrow. By ritualizing their stories as part of God's story, the pastoral minister will help the sick, their families and friends, as well as the Christian community to understand the place of God in suffering. This understanding may also help the sick to find meaning in suffering.

Chapter one discusses in detail the healing effects of bedside storytelling and listening. In this chapter, hospital bedside listening is presented as an important aspect of showing hospitality to the sick. Hospitality here refers to the act of providing the sick with the freedom or the opportunity to relate their stories and experiences. Hospitality also involves sharing the patients' stories with the worshipping community for better understanding. Chapter one also acknowledges what the sick can offer to the worshipping community. The sick can be sacrament for the community at large in that they mediate God's grace to the community. The sick teach the meaning of suffering. In this first chapter also, the act of helping the sick find meaning in suffering will be explored.

Because this research project has much to do with interpersonal discussions with patients, chapter two discusses the skills necessary to achieve meaningful conversation with the sick. Chapter two also includes some relevant theories, reflections, and commentaries by communication experts. This chapter introduces the concepts of rapport building, listening skills, and the recognition of sensory preferences in conversation. The sensory preference of a person according to Neuro-Linguistic Programming (NLP), simply posits that an individual has a preferred sense (though certainly not exclusive) for experiencing the world, i.e., acquiring, retaining and expressing information. The three primary senses are sight (visual), hearing (auditory), and feeling (kinesthetic).

Chapter three explains in detail how to apply some of the communication skills in a hospital context. This chapter also presents ways to connect and converse with hospital patients, to encourage confidence in the chaplain or pastoral minister so that significant stories are shared with the chaplain or pastoral minister. There will be examples of such conversations between the preacher and the patient as I have experienced them in some hospitals. This chapter also will include suggestions for documenting the patient's story after conversation as well as the ethical implications involved.

Chapter four explains the steps a preacher takes in preparing homilies for patients, starting from the encounter at bedside to writing a homily that will address the problems of the sick. Preparing these homilies involves taking into account the Biblical text and the encounter with the patient or the story the preacher has heard at bedside. Though some of these steps have been generally explained in chapter two, there is need to organize or apply them step by step as a clear guide for the preacher. These steps also can be used for Sunday liturgies and for daily liturgical preaching.

Chapter five describes the process for evaluating the effectiveness of some sample homilies. The evaluation involves a test of the effectiveness of the sermons preached using patients' stories. In order to test whether the integration of patients' stories in sermons makes a difference in how preaching is received by patients in a hospital setting, three homilies without patients' stories and three with patients' stories are used. Sermons preached without patients' stories refer to those sermons which focus on a Biblical text and may or may not use stories that do not come from hospital patients. Those sermons preached with patients' stories integrate their stories with a Biblical text.

The method of testing is with questionnaires designed to provide opportunities to patients to express how they felt about the homilies. Apart from using questionnaires, face-to-face conversations between the pastoral minister and patients are also provided. Their reactions are used to evaluate the sample homilies to determine whether or not the inclusion of patients' stories and experiences are of significant importance to the effectiveness of sermons preached in health care settings.

Chapter One

Hospital Bedside Listening as True Hospitality to the Sick

HOSPITALITY, NOT HOSTILITY

When the word "hospitality" is mentioned, we seem to think more about taking care of visitors or strangers who have lost or left their own homes, communities, and countries for other places. Hospitality to strangers can also apply to our brothers and sisters who have lost their health and have become estranged or alienated from us due to illness. However, everyone deserves hospitality, "especially those who struggle with loneliness and who are seeking warm and accepting relationships."[1] Hospitality in the health care setting includes giving the sick the freedom or the opportunity to express themselves and to be listened to. Unfortunately, in some cases, true hospitality has been found wanting in many of our communities and in the world at large.

In his book *Reaching Out*, Henri Nouwen laments that the world is full of strangers who have become more subject to hostility than to hospitality. Though there are instances of true hospitality to strangers, Nouwen points out that there are evidences of people greeting strangers with fearful aggression, instead of offering them an open and hospitable space and reaching out to them with love. Nouwen identifies the causes of this unfriendly attitude toward strangers as fear, suspicion, and ignorance of what the stranger can offer in our communities.[2]

The sick are not free from this unfriendly attitude. In her book the *Alchemy of Illness*, Kat Duff, speaking specifically for the sick, states a similar problem regarding unfriendliness which some sick people may face in their communities. Sometimes, the attitudes of the healthy toward the sick are negative because of the chronic nature of the sickness or ignorance with the mechanics of illness and with the feelings of the sick. Writing from experience, as someone who had suffered from a long lasting illness, Duff argues that as a result of the prejudice, suspicion, and blame that follows illness, many people living with disabling diseases lose the support of family and friends.[3]

As an alien in a foreign land, I know how important it is to feel accepted. In reaching out to our fellow human beings, especially to the sick who are estranged from their families and friends due to illness, we must be hospitable. Certainly, the sick are in need of our warm and accepting relationships. But how, exactly, do we do it? Nouwen argues that it involves creating "the free and friendly space"[4] in which those who are estranged can feel free, more cared for, loved, and accommodated as members of our religious and social communities. Such a free and friendly space can bring about transformation and fuller understanding. It is by so doing that the host or the pastoral minister recognizes the contributions of the stranger or the sick in the community.

ACTIVE/INTENTIONAL LISTENING TO WHAT THE SICK HAVE TO OFFER

Duff observes that the healthy, including health workers and pastors, can be ignorant of what the sick can offer to the community. It is wrong for the host to assume that the stranger has nothing to offer. On the contrary, the sick are in possession of gifts, which they are eager to make available to their hosts.[5]

The relationship between the host and the stranger should be seen as reciprocal. In order to gain from the experiences of the sick, it is necessary for the pastoral minister to clear any prejudices against the sick. This unbiased attitude toward the sick will bring about more openness. Also, the pastoral minister should be ready to apply significant listening skills in every encounter with the patient. In this sense, hospitality is not only expressed by being present at their bedsides, but also by being ready to listen to their stories and share their emotions, feelings, and thoughts.

Through such intentional listening to what the sick have to say about their experiences, valuable information may be gained by the listener about difficult and mysterious illnesses. As Duff recommends, it is necessary for those who are living with dreaded illnesses to be allowed to tell their whole stories, and to relate to others their feelings and experiences. Such information has been useful for research and has resulted in breakthroughs for curing diseases.[6] Also, we shall consider other contributions the sick make to the community, especially in liturgical contexts.

FROM HOSPITALITY TO FINDING MEANING IN SUFFERING: VICTOR FRANKL'S LOGOTHERAPY AND A PERSONAL INCIDENT

Finding meaning in suffering refers to the ability to find reasons either to hope for survival or to cope with illness. The sick can be assisted to find meaning in their suffering conditions through hospitality. In *Man's Search for Meaning*, Victor Frankl tells a graphic personal story of what happened to him and his fellow Jews in the Nazi concentration camps of World War II.[7] Writing from personal experience, he reveals the horrific hostility and aggression they experienced in terms of physical and mental torture, and ultimately the gassing of millions of fellow Jews to death.

In using Victor Frankl's experiences, I am not suggesting that life in the death camps was equal to the suffering of patients with chronic or terminal illnesses. However, we can say that suffering is common to both situations. In a situation of suffering, especially in humanly-inflicted suffering, the sick ask many questions in attempt to understand their pain-filled suffering. From personal experience, it is natural for a person undergoing suffering to seek for meaning. How does the pastoral minister assist the sick in finding meaning in their suffering?

Frankl tells the story of how he played the host in prison by creating space for some of his fellow prisoners to tell their stories to find meaning in their suffering. He applied what he calls logotherapy. Logotherapy is a meaning-oriented psychotherapeutic technique through which Frankl listened to the prisoners' stories and helped them find reasons to keep on hoping and clinging to life until the day of liberation.[8] Even when a typhoid epidemic broke out in the camp, many of those who contracted the disease, including Frankl himself, survived because he had reached out to motivate them to find meaning in their lives or reasons to keep on living.[9] In Frankl's opinion, many of the prisoners who did not make it to liberation would have survived if they had someone to listen to them and assist them find meaning in suffering.

Frankl was a prisoner himself suffering the same hardship as others, but his ability to open up the *free and friendly space*, to listen and be listened to, helped him and the other prisoners. This indicates that hospitality to the sick is a mutual engagement that helps not only the stranger but also the host. Like the prisoners in Frankl's story, many sick people need somebody to be at their bedsides to listen to their stories and apply the same logotherapy which Frankl recommends. Frankl's method of helping those suffering find meaning and hope has been resourceful to me in reaching out to my patients.

Logotherapy may or may not remove the physical suffering of the patient but can help the patient change his attitude toward his suffering condition.[10]

I recall my encounter with an accident victim with whom I tested my ability to help a person in a suffering condition find meaning and move on with life. A young man in his twenties, Joey (not his real name), was driving home from a party with his friends when he lost control of his car and crashed into a heavily wooded area. He had been driving under the influence of alcohol. Two of Joey's friends died in this accident while he was paralyzed from the waist down. He was brought to one of the hospitals where I was on call for sacramental ministry. When I entered Joey's room, I saw a sad and troubled young man who did not want to see anybody. I tried to present myself as a friend who was concerned about his condition. After greeting him and introducing myself to him, I commented about his sad mood and asked him to talk to me about what was going on. My asking gave him the opportunity to speak. He related how he felt about the accident and also his intention to take his own life because he blamed himself for the death of his two close friends.

Joey did not find any reason why he should continue living as a paralyzed man who would always be confined to a wheel chair. He would not be able to do things that he used to do for himself, but would instead need somebody else to help him. The worst thing for Joey was that he had a beautiful girl friend and feared she was going to abandon him for another. He couldn't imagine his girlfriend in the arms of another man while he languished in a wheelchair. He asked, "What is the sense in continuing with this life?" Initially, I was confused as to what to tell him, but I recalled Frankl's method of logotherapy. Consequently, I first thanked Joey for telling me his story. I told him that I did not blame him for feeling the way he felt or even for planning to take his life.

I inquired of him what he had been doing for a living before the accident, and he told me that he was a shoe designer. I asked him if he loved this job and would like to continue it, even while in his wheelchair, and he answered yes. When I asked him if there was anything he had wished to accomplish in his job before the accident, he responded with his plan of developing many new shoe designs. I sought Joey's opinion about still continuing to develop those designs while in his wheelchair. He reacted by nodding his head in acceptance and told me that it was a good idea, which had never occurred to him. I expressed that I, too, was saddened by the death of his good friends, and at the same time, relieved that he had survived. I then asked Joey to reflect on why God had spared his life in the accident. I also wanted Joey to consider his feelings about continuing in his design work instead of taking his own life. While I did not make any decisions for him, I asked him to think about these issues and then let me know his feelings next time we would meet.

During my follow-up visit, Joey was looking much better. He thanked me for talking with him previously. He believed that I helped him see his condition in a different way which in turn helped him to drop his former plan of taking his own life. Another piece of good news was that his girlfriend had promised him that she was not going to abandon him because of his condition.

THE HEALING EFFECT OF STORYTELLING: THE TWO CASES OF JAN NEWHOUSE AND JIM

My encounters with many patients lead me to believe that isolation is one of the major problems of the sick. Richard Stone argues that the very act of sharing a story with friends, family members, and other human beings contradicts the depressing isolation that many of us experience in life.[11]

In *Moon Dance, Life through the Cancer Lens,* Jan Newhouse, acknowledges how the generous acts of hospitality from her husband and her daughter helped her not only to cope with her cancer but also to find a reason why she should keep fighting her cancer, at least until her daughter was old enough to live on her own.[12] When her husband and daughter listened to her share her experiences, she found wholeness from other aspects of their love and kindness. She asserts, "My husband was very supportive during my cancer, doing the grocery shopping, vacuuming the house, or holding and hugging me when I was feeling down. He's a very honest man and would not say things he didn't know to be true. . . ."[13] Newhouse was thinking of how she was going to leave this honest and loving husband without a wife and leave her tender daughter without a mother. Speaking about her feelings for her daughter, she asserted, "Although uncertainty rules the world of cancer, there was one certainty for me from the day of first diagnosis: I would do everything in my power to live until my young daughter was old enough to thrive on her own."[14]

In situations when illness may be terminal, gracious acts of hospitality to the sick can help them come to terms with their illnesses and achieve wholeness.[15] In *Dear Bradie*, pastoral minister Martha Brunell records an encounter with a patient, Jim, who in his forties had ALS (Amyotrophic Lateral Sclerosis), a fatal, probably fast moving, and progressive neuro-muscular disease. Not enough is known about the disease in medical science and there is yet no known cure.[16]

Though his illness was terminal, Jim had one major thing to accomplish that could give him fulfillment. He was concerned about his three year old daughter, Bradie. Jim feared she was too young to understand his great love for her or comprehend the dynamics of his terminal illness. Jim needed someone to give him the opportunity to tell his stories, which would be recorded for his daughter. For Jim to find some happiness or fulfillment in this situation of suffering, he needed to be able to tell his daughter how much he had loved her and for her to have something that could help her remember her father's love and presence in her life even when he was gone.[17]

In her pastoral encounter with Jim, Brunell understood Jim's concern and was able to offer Jim that friendly and free space. She listened to Jim express himself about his experiences and his life, even though he couldn't talk much, and she wrote for Jim a series of love letters for Bradie. Brunell's pastoral response helped Jim to come to terms with his ALS and to find wholeness in the face of on-coming death.

Hospitality from a pastor or health worker can help the sick achieve fulfillment and can also help family members to find meaning and to cope with their losses. Brunell's visits and her recording of Jim's story for his daughter not only helped Jim have a deep sense of wholeness and fulfillment, but also in the retelling of his story, Bradie would know more of her past. Again Brunell's intervention could also be a source of healing for Bradie in accepting the loss of her father. Brunnel's act of hospitality helped Jim find integration with his family and friends.

Jim's second wish and source of fulfillment was how to tell his story in such a way that could inform the public on what it means to live and die with ALS. His experiences with the disease helped other people learn more about ALS and how Jim successfully handled this terminal disease with knowledgeable and supportive pastoral care. With his generosity and sense of humor, Jim held on to life until he had exhausted all his feelings about the disease. All these accomplishments brought healing to Jim even as he was breathing his last breaths.

A similar experience of coming to terms with illness and accepting death with courage and fulfillment was narrated by Brunell in "Hibiscus Blaze." It is a true story of a woman named Irma and her family. Irma also suffered from ALS and was able to share significant meaning as her death approached simply because of the pastoral hospitality and acceptance offered her by Brunell as well as Irma's family.

SHARING THE PATIENT'S BEDSIDE STORY WITH THE WORSHIPING COMMUNITY

Hospitality to the sick, practiced by being present and offering the sick an opportunity to tell their stories, can also bring about a better understanding of how to relate with the sick. In line with Nouwen's argument, true hospitality can bring about re-creative community with the sick. By sharing their stories, the sick feel less alienation and estrangement from the community of the healthy. This positive result implies that the pastoral minister will not stop at listening to their stories; it also must involve the pastoral minister taking action. As indicated by James D. Whitehead and Evelyn Eaton Whitehead, the information gained by listening generates insight on how best we can respond to the needs of others.[18] With the insight gained after listening and reflecting, the pastoral minister responds by sharing the stories of the sick (while observing all the ethical rules of handling information and confidentiality of the sick) with the Christian community, especially in a liturgical context; for example, a sermon at a worship service.

Sharing a patient's story in liturgical celebration enhances the spirit of community.[19] In the sharing of stories, the healthy members of the worshipping community may be able to better understand the sick. By reducing prejudice, fear, and suspicion against the sick, the community may understand and accept them as brothers and sisters of the Lord's Table and receive the gifts the sick have to offer. These practices call to mind one of the things Jesus asked the sick to do after healing them of their illnesses, ". . . go and show yourself to the priest and make the offering for your cleansing prescribed by Moses as evidence to them" (Mark 1:44). Healing is completed when the sick have been integrated once more as part of the community.

However, due to their suffering conditions, the sick cannot come to the pastor to tell their stories; rather, the pastoral minister needs to take the initiative, as Jesus took the initiative, to come among them, listen to them, feel with them, and be their voice to the community. The pastoral minister needs to share their stories with the community in celebrating the Word and the Sacrament of the Eucharist. In the Word, the community hears or shares their stories, while in the Eucharist the sick become one with the community.

Patients may gain from the communal activity of the liturgy whether they are present physically or are watching the liturgy on closed circuit television. They may identify similarities in the stories of others who are or who were in similar suffering conditions. The ability of identifying similarities or to see aspects of one's own life in the stories of others can help the sick to draw strength and gain some solace and recognition. Above all, when a pastoral minister integrates the real stories of patients into his sermons, he can make it easier for other patients to identify with the situation and thereby improve the chances that the gospel message will sound more meaningful and relevant. Adults learn best when what is being learned is both meaningful and relevant.

Hospitality involves interpersonal communication. In the next two chapters, we shall examine the communication skills involved in interpersonal communication. We shall first discuss these communication skills as they occur in our day to day conversations before applying them to the hospital context.

NOTES

1. Verlyn D. Verbrugge, *The NIV Topical Study Bible: Hospitality* (Grand Rapids, Michigan: Zondervan Bible Publishers, 1989), 1413.
2. Henri Nouwen, *Reaching Out: The Movements of the Spiritual Life* (New York: Doubleday Publishing Company, 1975), 47.
3. Kat Duff, *The Alchemy of Illness* (New York: Bell Tower, 1993), 30.
4. Nouwen, 50.
5. Ibid., 61.
6. Duff, *The Alchemy of Illness*, 31.
7. Viktor E. Frankl, *Man's Search for Meaning* (New York: Pocket Books, 1984), 21.
8. Ibid, 120.
9. Frankl, 120.
10. Ibid, 136.
11. Richard Stone, *The Healing Art of Storytelling: A Sacred Journey of Personal Discovery* (New York: Author Choice Press, 2004), 3.
12. Jan Newhouse, *Moon Dance: Life through the Cancer Lens* (St. Louis, Missouri: Avery Publishing, 2004), 5.
13. Ibid., 15.
14. Ibid., 5.
15. 28.
16. Martha Brunell, "Hibiscus Blaze," An unpublished Article on Pastoral Care of ALS Patient, St. Louis.
17. Martha A. Brunell: *In Dear Bradie: A Story of Life with ALS,* narrated, recorded and produced by Douglas D. Cripe, 2006, CD recording.
18. James D. Whitehead and Evelyn Eaton Whitehead, *Methods in Ministry: Theological Reflection and Christian Ministry* (Kansas City, Missouri: Sheed and Ward, 1995), 16.
19. Stone, 13.

Chapter Two

Interpersonal Conversation

In chapter one, we discussed the importance of giving free and friendly space to the sick in order that they might express themselves and be listened to. Also, we emphasized the importance of moving their stories from bedside to pulpit. This movement of patients' stories from bedside to pulpit has much to do with interpersonal discussion between the pastoral ministers and patients. In this chapter, we discuss the views of some communication experts on what goes on when two or more people are exchanging information.

WHY DO WE CONVERSE OR COMMUNICATE?

In *Making Connections,* Charles T. Meadow helps us to understand one of the most common reasons why people communicate. Communication has many purposes, but the major one is to transfer or to exchange information.[1] We are concerned here with interpersonal exchange of information which takes place between two or more people. Interpersonal communication is a necessary social act which helps to define us as human beings.[2] We need to come together with others to interact and to exchange ideas either as members of families, or as friends at work, or as members of communities. Without interpersonal connection with others, we cannot exist because we cannot do without the support of other people in our lives.

Commenting on the importance and the social nature of human interaction, Harlene Anderson asserts, "One of the most important features of life is conversation. We are in continuous conversation with each other and with ourselves. Through conversation we form and reform our life experiences and events; we create and recreate our meanings and understandings; and we construct and reconstruct realities and ourselves."[3] Whether in good times or in hard times, we need the support of other people. According to Nicholas Boothman, through body language, gestures, facial expressions, and words of others, we are strengthened in difficult times and our good times become more enjoyable.[4] Many people have become frustrated in life simply because they have few relations and friends to talk to, and sometimes their life experiences become a burden they cannot carry alone.

My interactions with patients in hospitals help me realize how important our need is to support each other, especially in the difficult moments of our lives. In Scripture, Luke's gospel (8:26-39) presents the storm rising while Jesus was in the same boat with his disciples. Jesus not only calmed the storm but also gave his disciples his support. The storm of illness or sorrow must one day come to all of us. In such a situation, the burden is lighter when we have the support of one another.

THE COOPERATIVE PRINCIPLE IN INFORMATION EXCHANGE

For information exchange to be accomplished well, communicators (speakers and listeners) must follow the cooperative principle which guides how people speak and interpret. The cooperative principle requires that talk should be directed as required. For Karen Tracy, conversation is seen as "a cooperative activity." It can be compared to a soccer game which demands cooperative team work as all the players are expected to follow the rules for a meaningful game.[5]

USING THE PROPER REFERENCE TERMS IN CONVERSATION

In addressing another person or group of persons, it is necessary for the communicator to know the proper reference term or terms to use for a partner or partners in conversation. Tracy points out that using the appropriate terms in conversation makes a difference and could have some implications for speakers and their targets.[6] That is to say that when the appropriate titles or terms are used to address a person or a group in an interpersonal encounter, the response will be more cordial and friendly than when a less appropriate reference term is used.

Tracy talks about personal address, which refers to "the label we give to terms used to refer to a person in his or her presence."[7] Some people may not like to be addressed by their formal first names but may prefer the diminutive version of their first names (Katy instead of Kathleen or Bill instead of William). It is not that such people would be offended if called by their real first names, but they may prefer their nicknames. They also respond better when called by their nicknames.

Tracy also indicates that the use of a more acceptable kinship name is very important in interpersonal communication. Kinship names refer to names given to mothers (Mama, Mom), fathers (Dad, Popi), grandparents, aunts, and uncles.[8] Cultural differences can also determine which of the above terms can be used in addressing people. When I first came to the United States, I used the term "Mom" to address most of the elderly women whom I visited in the hospitals because I felt they were old enough to be my mother. I was later advised by one of my supervisors to better use the term "Ma'am" for adult women. The fact was that some of the women did not like my calling them "Mom" because we were not biologically related, and some of them felt old when they observed a person of my age calling them mom. In Nigeria, using the word "Mom" to address a woman of childbearing age is considered an honor. Most women in Nigeria would appreciate it.

The use of the proper or acceptable term also applies when a communicator is addressing a group. The identity of any group needs to be considered and respected. Using a culturally unacceptable reference term to talk to a group of people could bring about negative interpersonal effects. For example, one Nigerian Navy officer who was trained in the United States was asked by the Nigerian military government to come home to be the governor of one of the states in the country. It was part of the protocol for the new governor of a state to address a group of traditional rulers in the state. Traditional rulers are from royal families and are always greeted with respect. They are seen as the upholders of the culture of the land and as fathers of the people. The new governor started his address by greeting the traditional rulers with "hi guys." In Nigeria, using the word "guys" is foreign and it is regarded as a very casual greeting, more suitable for teenagers in high school. The traditional leaders were unhappy. They expressed their dissatisfaction with the new governor.

INTERPRETING IDENTITY THROUGH CONVERSATION

Apart from information exchange, people reveal identity through conversing with others. The communicator's style of talking can reveal more about his identities in terms of nationality, age, profession, and social class.[9] Having resided in the United States for about seven years, I am still identified as a foreigner when people hear me speak. They ask, "Where are you from? You have an accent. Are you from Africa?" When I tell them that I am from Nigeria, they say, "No wonder! We can tell by the way you speak." I speak the same English language as others, but my accent introduces me first, even before I tell people about my background and my nationality.

MAKING MEANING OUT OF INTERPERSONAL CONVERSATION

In writing about the meaning-making process in interpersonal conversation, Tracy posits that in any talk, the utterance of the speaker, whether a word or a phrase or a long statement, is what creates meaning. For her, our utterances are linguistic expressions but also units of social life.[10] An utterance like "hello," could be a response to another utterance. For example, I visited a patient in one of the hospitals and greeted him, "Hello, Mr. Smith." He replied, "Hello, Pastor." Tracy suggests that an utterance like "hello" has two levels of meaning. The first meaning comes from the *content* while the second meaning comes from the *context*. The content refers to the conventional meaning or the literal meaning of the word or phrase. When I said hello to Mr. Smith as I entered his room, my greeting was friendly and he replied in a similar friendly tone. This greeting is the first level of meaning.

The second level of meaning is what Tracy calls the interactional meaning which is determined by the context in which the hello was said.[11] I remember my conversation with a woman inside the chapel of one of the hospitals. We were talking about the current events, about the high crime rate in some neighborhoods in the city of St. Louis. At the beginning of our discussion, everything seemed normal until she started talking about how her ex-husband used to physically abuse her. In telling me how her ex-husband used to punch her as if she were a punching bag, she became very emotional and started raising her voice. Because she was raising her voice, I started speaking in a low tone, "hell-oooh, hell-oooh" with the second syllable drawn out. The prolongation of the syllable gave it a different meaning. It was not a greeting in this context, but an effort to call my conversation partner's attention to the sacredness of the chapel.

INTERPERSONAL COMMUNICATION AS A PROCESS OF RENDERING HELP

As we saw at the beginning of this chapter, one of the major reasons why people engage in interpersonal communication is to exchange information. People have different goals for exchanging information. For pastoral purposes, interpersonal communication is a process of helping someone in need. According to Eugene W. Kelly, helping is here understood to mean "an interpersonal communication process in which one person is responding to another so as to facilitate and foster the personal growth, welfare and problem-solving of the other."[12]

The ultimate goal in looking at interpersonal communication as a process of rendering help is for the communicator to contribute to the wellbeing of those who may in one way or another need help. For interpersonal communication to be really helpful, it has to involve some communication skills.

RAPPORT BUILDING

Rapport building is very important in human communication. Good rapport assures a more fruitful conversation between two or more people. In *How To Make People Like You in 90 Seconds or Less,* Boothman explains rapport in these words.

> Rapport is the establishment of common ground or a comfort zone where two or more people can mentally join together. When you have rapport, each of you brings something to the interaction— attentiveness, warmth, a sense of humor, for example—and each brings something back: empathy, sympathy, maybe a couple of great jokes. Rapport is the lubricant that allows social exchanges to flow smoothly.[13]

Jane Jorgenson agrees with Boothman that rapport is an aspect of interpersonal relationship that is shared or jointly experienced. The advantage of establishing rapport is the other person's positive acceptance and happiness in speaking with his conversation partner. When the skills of rapport are not applied, attention may be more difficult to achieve. Jorgensen also agrees that rapport could facilitate cooperation, especially in interviews for data collection.[14] In *The Worst Is Over*, Judith Acosta and Judith Simon Prager state that "without rapport, effective communication is simply not possible."[15] They explain rapport as establishing a firm foundation before building a house that can stand. In a situation of rendering help or responding to the needs of someone, if the communicator or helper does not first establish enough rapport, his conversational partner or helpee will not have enough trust to reveal personal stories.[16] Kelly supports the claim of Acosta and Prager, positing that rapport is basic to effective interpersonal communication. Helping is not possible unless there is a working relationship between the helper and the helpee, i.e., sufficient mutual acceptance to allow the process to proceed in a useful manner. As time goes on and the relationship develops, simple acceptance usually blossoms into trust and respect.[17]

From my hospital encounters with patients, I believe that when a strong rapport is not established, most patients will not reveal how they actually feel. Many of them may say that they are feeling okay while their facial expressions, voice tones, and body positioning tell a different story. However, when enough rapport has been established, I am often surprised at the tremendous amount of information they share about what is going on in their lives in connection with their illnesses.

Boothman establishes a systemic way of establishing rapport, though he accepts that sometimes rapport just happens all by itself, as if by chance, while at other times the communicator has to establish it. Boothman believes that as one greets people, one's ability to establish rapport will depend on four skills: attitude, ability to "synchronize" certain aspects of behavior like body language and voice tone, conversational skills, and ability to discover which sense or senses (visual, auditory or kinesthetic) the other person relies on when receiving and presenting information.[18]

Jorgensen seems to disagree with Boothman on how easily rapport may be established. She asserts, "My personal associations with the word 'rapport' are complex. As a student of communication, I am intrigued by the richness of its relational implications and yet doubtful of settling on a mode of investigation of rapport that would fully allow for its emergent systemic nature."[19] She accepts that the discovery of shared identity, such as gender can contribute to the growth of rapport, but she finds it difficult to explain or predict which shared identities would come into play in a given encounter.[20] Boothman believes that if there is a situation in which no shared interest is present, rapport could be established by design. Boothman identifies three different types of rapport necessary for interpersonal communication. These are rapport by nature, by chance, and by design.[21]

RAPPORT BY NATURE

Rapport by nature suggests common ground with some people due to our natural connections with them. For example, from birth, we have depended on emotional contact, signs, and symbols from our parents, peers, teachers, and friends. People with common interests have natural rapport.[22] No one needs to establish a fresh rapport before communicating with parents, brothers, and sisters. The rapport is already established by natural affiliation.

RAPPORT BY CHANCE

Rapport also could be by chance. This kind of rapport may happen when someone travels to a country in which his or her language is not ordinarily spoken. All of a sudden, the person hears someone from his own country who speaks his language. Both of them may quickly become friendly, and this friendship is by chance because the common language becomes a common ground that brings the two of them together to start interacting with one another.[23]

The first friendships I made when I first came to the United States began in a shopping mall. When I heard someone speaking my native language, I turned and spoke to the man in this language and he responded. Immediately, we became friendly and exchanged phone numbers, and the friendship developed to the extent that now I feel part of his family. Of course, when rapport by nature and rapport by chance are not implied, rapport by design can be applied, especially in a first time meeting.

RAPPORT BY DESIGN

Sometimes, a communicator may not have time for rapport to happen naturally. In such a situation, the communicator needs to do something to create common ground with his conversational partner. Rapport by design is established by deliberately altering one's behavior, just for a short time, in order to become like the other person. This will involve applying the right attitude, the art of synchronizing, applying conversational skills, and finding the person's sensory preferences.[24]

THE SKILLS OF ESTABLISHING RAPPORT

Acquiring the skills of building rapport is very necessary in order for there to be a more effective connection between the communicator (the helper) and a conversational partner (the helpee), especially when the communicator is encountering a partner for the first time. In order for a conversational partner to accept the communicator and be ready to talk with him, the communicator must present himself well.

The first impression matters in any conversation. If the communicator creates a proper impression within some seconds of a new meeting, he creates awareness that he is friendly, trustworthy, and sincere. The ability to create the right impression enhances rapport building that can make the meeting more cordial.[25] The following skills can help the communicator establish rapport that could lead to a friendly conversational relationship.

THE GREETING

It is natural and proper for conversational partners to greet each other during a meeting, especially when the meeting is taking place for the first time. In

How To make People Like You in 90 Seconds or Less, Boothman proposes five parts of an effective greeting. The five parts are Open—Eye—Beam—Hi—Lean. These five parts of greeting are to take place within a few seconds of contact.

Open

Open body language is very important in communication. In his text *Communicator Style*, Norton Robert recommends a body movement that is expansive, unreserved, extroverted, and approach oriented.[26] When the communicator meets with someone the first time, his body language should be open. The communicator's heart has to be aimed at the person he is meeting. He should not fold his arms. If possible, he should unbutton his coat or jacket.[27] These examples suggest openness.

Body language (posture, expressions, and gestures) forms more than half of what people respond to when they are making up their minds about the communicator or the person meeting them.[28] Body language should signal cooperation, agreement, willingness, enthusiasm, and approval. In *How To Talk to Anyone*, Leil Lowndes asserts, "The way you look and the way you move is more than 80 percent of someone's first impression of you. Not one word need be spoken."[29] Lowndes emphasizes that when the communication partner looks at the communicator, the partner immediately starts to form impressions about the communicator. The effect of such early impressions forms the foundation for the whole relationship.

Eye

Eye contact is the second aspect of the greeting process. Eye behavior, especially a direct eye gaze, signals readiness to interact. Eye contact also projects involvement. Virginia P. Richmond and James C. McCroskey posit that in American culture, it is difficult to establish eye contact with someone, even with a stranger, without some level of interaction.[30] With eye contact, a simple interaction of smiling at another person or nodding of the head is expected.

The communicator needs to take the lead in making eye contact by looking directly into the eyes of the new person. Boothman states that looking away from the new person sends the wrong signal or may even suggest lack of interest. The communicator's eye contact should make his partner feel that the communicator has a positive attitude.[31] Lowndes supports this idea by talking of "epoxy eyes." The epoxy eye technique is the act of looking at your target with full concentration and interest. "When you use epoxy eyes, it sends out signals of interest blended with complete confidence in yourself."[32]

Unlike Boothman, Lowndes warns that there should be caution. "Don't overdo it or you could come across as arrogant and brazen."[33] In some cultures, too much eye contact could be seen as harassment, especially when it makes the other person feel uncomfortable. Roger E. Axtell reveals that in Japan, Korea, and Thailand, prolonged direct eye contact is not acceptable because it is considered impolite and even intimidating.[34]

Beam

Eye contact is followed with a beaming smile which should reflect the communicator's positive attitude. To send a message of friendliness and sincerity to others, the communicator also needs to take the lead in smiling while looking directly into the eyes of the new person.[35] Lowndes believes that a big warm smile is an asset when meeting someone for the first time but suggests that the smile should not come too quickly in order for it to look credible. She suggests that the delay should be probably less than a second.[36] When the smile is beamed, the recipient or recipients will have the impression that the big warm smile is special and for them.

Hi

The communicator should be the first to say "Hi or "Hello" to the new person and should say it with pleasing tonality. While saying "Hi" or "Hello," the communicator should also be the first to identify himself and mention his name.[37] It could go this way, "Hi, my name is John." By taking the lead in revealing his name or identity, the communicator has invited the other person to respond likewise. When the person responds with a name, the communicator now has information on how to refer to this person.

In some situations, the communicator may already know the name of the person before first meeting. While saying "Hi" or "Hello," the communicator should call the name of the other person. Calling the name of the other person could be presented in this way, "Hi, Mr. Peters. My name is John." Mentioning the correct name of the person helps to create a friendly feeling. Sometimes the communicator may need to ask the other person the best way to pronounce his name. Also, some people may prefer being called by a nickname derived from their formal names. The use of nicknames may enhance rapport.

Lean

In using open body language, the communicator should lean forward while introducing himself. The communicator's forward-leaning action can be an almost "imperceptible forward tilt" to very subtly indicate interest and openness to the person he has just met.[38] Richmond and McCrowskey believe that this forward leaning is one of those body behaviors that help to reduce distance and create intimacy between two conversational partners.[39] In some African cultures, leaning forward while greeting someone is a mark of respect, especially for a senior or someone of high reputation. Having performed the above initial introductory skills correctly, some physical contact or handshake between the communicator and the new person is likely to follow.

The Handshake

Most introductions should include a handshake if possible. Boothman advises that handshakes should be firm and respectful.[40] However, it may be better for the other person to determine the firmness of the handshake. In some cultures, especially in the Middle East and in some Asian cultures, people prefer a handshake with a gentle grip because a firm grip is regarded as a mark of aggression.[41]

The handshake usually follows the lean. Though the communicator should initiate a handshake with the new person, he must be careful about differences in cultures. In American culture, for instance, a man may not be the first to initiate a handshake with a woman. It is better to allow a woman to initiate the handshake. If the woman does not initiate it, the communicator should move on with other rapport-building skills.

Applying Right Attitude

Applying a useful attitude determines the quality of the communicator's relationship. When meeting someone for the first time, the communicator can be supportive, enthusiastic, inquiring, helpful, and engaging. The communicator's posture, movements, and expression will speak volumes about him even before he opens his mouth. On the other hand, useless attitudes like being angry, sarcastic, disrespectful, rude, and anxious can ruin rapport.[42] To encourage application of useful attitude by the communicator, T. Dean Thomlison writes of mutual sharing of selves in a face-to-face encounter. Mutual sharing entails being considerate along with a mutual attempt to develop common ground. In mutual sharing, the communicator must not try to gain power or control over the other person.[43] Any attempt to control a partner in conversation should be resisted as this control spoils genuineness, confidence, and trust in interpersonal relationship.

Ability to Synchronize

One of the most effective ways of establishing rapport is the ability to synchronize another person's behavior. Synchronicity may involve the communicator doing what his partner does; the communicator acts like the other until the other person finds it more interesting to be with him.[44] It is a connecting or adapting device that makes a person see his conversational partner connected to him. Synchronizing is a way to make a person become open, relaxed, and happy to be with the other. This synchronization can be done within seconds of meeting the other person. Boothman clarifies, suggests that synchronicity is different from being insincere or being phony.

Synchronicity in interpersonal communication may involve matching voice tones, facial expression, body language, body posture, and particular gestures. For example, if the communicator meets someone who speaks to him in a low tone, in order to match, the communicator may also respond or speak in a low tone. For someone who speaks loudly, the communicator synchronizes by speaking in a loud tone. If the other person smiles, the communicator follows and smiles; if the person withdraws the smile, the communicator withdraws his own. All these help to enhance rapport. The essence of establishing rapport is to have a good conversation with the new person.

CONVERSATION WITH THE NEW PERSON

Conversation time comes after the communicator has met someone new and within seconds has carried out the introductory process as described above and has established some level of rapport. Conversation can also be a remarkable way to continue establishing more rapport and strengthening the bonds of friendship. Conversation comes in two parts: talking and listening. It may also involve asking discussion-inducing questions and engaging in active listening.[45]

TALKING AND QUESTIONING

In starting a conversation, the communicator should allow the other person or client to start talking to reveal some areas of his or her interest while the communicator listens and synchronizes. In some situations, the communicator may start by asking the client a discursive question that could encourage the other person into a conversation. Boothman calls questions the "spark plugs of conversation."[46] As spark plugs set off the car engine, questions trigger the client to talk and give detailed information about areas of concern. In *Conversation, Language, and Possibilities*, Harlene Anderson agrees with Boothman and also asserts, "Questions are the core of any interview or therapy conversation. They facilitate or hinder the story a client wants to tell."[47]

Anderson goes on to explain that in asking questions, the communicator needs to ask relevant questions. Irrelevant questions can make clients feel the communicator did not hear or understand what was said. Irrelevant questions may make the clients feel unimportant, insulted, and also hinder them from telling their stories further. Anderson also recommends asking questions from the position of "not-knowing" what could be the answer the client is going to give to the question. She asserts,

> Questions from this (not-knowing) position help a client tell, clarify, and expand on a story; open up new avenues and explore what is known or not-known; they help a therapist learn about and avoid misconceptions of the *said* and the *not-yet-said.* In turn, each question leads to an elaboration of descriptions and explanations; each question leads to another question—a process of continuing questioning that provides springboards of a dialogical process.[48]

Anderson calls such questions *conversational questions* because they invite the client to talk *with* the communicator or therapist. In asking conversational questions, there may be need for the communicator to precede a question with an open statement or a rapport-inducing statement which encourages the other person to talk. The best rapport-inducing statement is a statement that is related to what you have in common with the person.[49] For example, "I love your shirt." "What beautiful weather today." Such open statements could encourage a person to make a comment even before a discursive question is asked.

Boothman points out that there are two types of questions: those that open people up and those that close them down. Open questions request an explanation and thus require the other person to do the talking. Closed questions elicit "yes" or "no" responses.[50] Anderson, in agreement with Boothman, advises asking the right question in order for the other person to give the right information. Anderson also believes that in the situation of therapy, the client expects the communicator to ask the right question.[51] Purdy and Borisoff agree with Anderson and also recommend that the tone of voice used in asking questions has a lot to do with how the question is received.[52] The questions should be fashioned in a way that could help the other person or client to express himself or herself freely and fully.

To ask an open question which would generate conversation, Boothman suggests starting with one of these conversation-generating words: *Who?*

When? Why? What? Where? How? Starting a question with any of these words demands an explanation, an opinion, or a feeling from the conversation partner.[53] Here are some examples of how to use these conversation-generating words: "How do you feel about your illness?" "What is your doctor saying about the cause of this illness?" "Why do you think that God does not love or care about you?"

The advantage of using these words is to make a faster connection and to enable the other person to start talking. Another way to bring forth more information is to use some sensory words like *see, feel,* and *tell.* Sensory words can boost these conversation- generators and can also give the other person the opportunity to bring forth more information.[54] "How do you *feel* about your family?" "When do you *see* your dream coming true?" "*Tell* me your impression about God in connection with what is happening to you."

While conversation is going on, the communicator should try to avoid using closing-down words in asking questions. Closing-down words include: "Are you . . . ?" "Do you . . . ?" "Have you . . . ?" They make rapport-inducing conversations more difficult because they elicit one word answers of "yes" or "no."[55] Using closing-down words, may require another question in order to get the type of answer or information the communicator wants.

LISTENING

Interpersonal communication involves both talking and listening. As Boothman suggests, listening is the other side of the conversation coin.[56] Listening is as important as speaking. Purdy and Borisoff observe that for most of Western civilization, speaking has been considered more important than listening. Listeners were recognized, but seen more as helping the speaker achieve his or her own purposes. Purdy and Borisoff observe that people have been given awards throughout Western history for being great and eloquent speakers, but not for being great listeners.[57] However, the impression that speaking is more important than listening is changing. People have come to realize that both speaking and listening are roads to success. A speaker would not succeed if there were no listeners.

LISTENING SKILLS

Listening can provide enormous power to bring about a successful interaction between people in personal and professional conditions.[58] For listening to be fruitful, the communicator must observe the following skills.

Listening with Interest

Effective listening demands that the communicator demonstrate to the other person that he is truly interested in what the other person is saying. The key to being an active listener lies in making a sincere effort to absorb what the other person is saying and feeling.[59] This could be why Anderson sees listening as "attending to, interacting with, responding to, and trying to learn about a client's story and its perceived importance."[60]

Boothman, however, differentiates listening from hearing. Active listening is an attempt to grasp, understand, feel the emotion that motivates talk, and response with appropriate feedback. A person could be hearing what the other person is saying without truly paying attention, especially when the listener is doing something else that shows that he or she is not paying attention to the speaker.

Listening and Giving Proper Response

Anderson believes that listening and hearing go hand-in-hand and cannot be separated. She emphasizes the responsive nature of listening by talking about "responsive-active listening-hearing" or the act of inviting clients to tell us how they feel about a particular issue or what could be their major concerns.[61] Inviting a client to express himself requires proper response or feedback from the therapist or listener. Proper response or feedback is easier given when the therapist is not only listening, but also hearing clearly what the client is saying.

In the words of Dennis M. Kratz and Abby Robinson Kratz, "Feedback refers to any message sent by the listener to the speaker either during or after the speaker's presentation."[62] The listener's action or response may encourage or discourage the speaker from communicating with the listener. It could take the form of nodding the head to show that the listener is listening attentively or conversely of looking away from the speaker to show that the listener is either bored or distracted or not paying attention. A good listener not only should be conscious of the importance of giving feedback but also be able to apply encouraging feedback.[63]

Listening and Contributing

The skills of listening also involve listening with the eyes, listening with the body, nodding one's head, looking at the person and encouraging the other person verbally.[64] The above actions show that the listener is part of the conversation or dialogue. Listening involves the contribution of both the person talking and the person listening. Anderson agrees with the above claim in these words:

> Responsive-active listening-hearing does not mean just sitting back and doing nothing. It does not mean that a therapist cannot say anything, offer an idea, or express an opinion. Nor does it mean that it is just a technique. Responsive-active listening-hearing is a natural therapist manner and attitude that communicates and demonstrates sincere interest, respect, and curiosity.[65]

Leslie A. Baxter and Barbara M. Montgomery seem to be saying the same thing by emphasizing respect for the voice of the other when they assert, "Critical to 'good conversation' is respect for the voice of the other without forcing the other to share one's viewpoint."[66] Conversation should be dialogical because it involves the contribution of both the person talking and the person listening. John Shorter in *Conversational Realities* calls it "joint action."[67] Joint action does not mean that the speaker and the listener should be talking at the same time or that the listener should interrupt the speaker at intervals while still talking. It means that the roles of both the speaker and the listener are equally needed for a meaningful conversation to take place.

Verbal contributions of the listener could come at intervals or when needed, in any of these ways, "You are saying the truth." "I heard what you said." Nonverbal contributions from a listener could be nodding of the head, looking directly at the speaker, smiles, postures that indicate attentiveness, facial expressions, and gestures[68] like a thumb's up to show acceptance and to congratulate the speaker.

Being Careful with Giving Advice

When someone is listening to another person tell his story, there is the temptation to start giving advice. Purdy and Borisoff strongly recommend avoiding giving advice or making a decision for the client. A listener's advice originates from the listener's personal experiences and may not be appropriate for another person. Moreover, giving advice may make the client or family members depend on the listener for answers. Purdy and Borisoff rather recommend empowering the client.[69] Let the client find his or her own solution based on his or her own experiences.

Purdy and Borisoff, however, do not totally rule out the importance of guidance, but it should be based on careful empathetic listening.[70] For example, as narrated in my encounter with Ken, who wanted to end his life, I did not advise him to take or not to take his life. I simply listened to him and helped him to see his condition in a different way. He later decided not to take his own life, not because I told him not to, but because I had helped him find meaning in continuing with life. My encounter with him helped him to make a healthier decision.

RECOGNIZING THE SENSORY PREFERENCES OF THE OTHER PERSON

Richard Bandler and John Grinder, founders of Neuro-Linguistic Programming (NLP), argue that every human person has a "favorite sense" through which he or she experiences the world and gets information. Bandler and Grinder classify people under the three senses which most people rely on: sight (visual), auditory (hearing), and kinesthetic (feeling). When a communicator discovers a person's favorite sense, it is easier to become more connected with that person and to open up the person's mind and heart.[71] Adapting Grinder and Bandler's ideas, Boothman believes that people recieve information by relying more on the senses of *sight*, *hearing*, and *feeling* or the way things *look*, *sound,* and *feel.*[72]

Boothman also posits that in relating information about experiences, people reveal what sense or senses they rely on. He calls these "explanatory styles."[73] As an example, we can look at the language of three soccer fans as they relate their experiences to their mother. John, Jane, and Jody attended a soccer competition at the stadium, and later their mother asks each to tell what they had experienced. John said, "Mom, I saw a huge number of people. When the goal was scored, I saw hundreds of people jumping up and down. Mom, you need to have seen this competition." John's response reveals that he is using more of picture words based on the sense of sight.

Jane's language was different. She said, "Mom, when our team scored the winning goal, everyone was shouting and the fans were beating the drums and singing songs of victory. Mom, you should have heard them." Jane is expressing her experiences of the competition based more on what she heard. Jane's expression shows that she relies more on the way things sound.

Jody said, "Mom, I felt so happy when our team scored the goal. The whole place was vibrating." Jody's information is based more on how she felt about the competition and the victory. Jody's expression shows that she relies more on the way things feel. The communicator has to listen carefully to recognize the sensory input of another. Using this information in personal, professional, or social dealings with a conversation partner can have a remarkable effect upon how a conversation partner responds.[74] In other words, when a communicator discovers the other person's sensory input, the communicator synchronizes the other person's use of words and expressions thereby more able to connect more and develop rapport faster.

The message the communicator gives to the other person is that they both have something in common.

In the next chapter, we shall apply all these communication skills to encountering patients in hospitals and getting information from them. The pastoral minister and other caregivers need these communication skills in order to gain the trust and confidence of their patients, so that they may reveal their personal stories. It is by telling their personal stories that the caregiver knows what service to provide to help the patient.

NOTES

1. Charles T. Meadow, *Making Connections: Communication through the Ages* (New York: Scarecrow Press Inc., 2002), 5.
2. Roberts Freed Bales, *Communication, Language, and Meaning: Communication in Small Groups* (New York: Basic Books, 1973), 208.
3. Harlene Anderson, *Conversation, Language, and Possibilities: A Postmodern Approach to Therapy* (New York: BasicBooks, 1997), xvii.
4. Nicholas Boothman, *How To Make People Like You in 90 Seconds or Less* (New York: Workman Publishing, 2000) 7.
5. Karen Tracy, *Everyday Talk: Building and Reflecting Identities* (New York: The Guildford Press 2002), 6.
6. Ibid., 46.
7. Ibid., 50.
8. Ibid., 50
9. Ibid., 7.
10. Ibid., 9.
11. Ibid., 8.
12. Eugene W. Kelly, *Effective Interpersonal Communication: A Manual for Skill Development* (Washington D.C.: University Press of America, 1979), 5.
13. Boothman, 19.
14. Jane Jorgensen, "Re-relationship Rapport in Interpersonal Settings," ed. Wendy Leeds Hurdwitz, *Social Approaches to Communication* (New York: Guildford Press, 1995), 155.
15. Judith Acosta and Judith Simon Prager, *The Worst Is Over: What To Say When Every Moment Counts* (San Diego, CA.: Jodere Group, 2003), 51.
16. Ibid.
17. Kelly, 5.
18. Boothman, 19.
19. Jorgensen, 155.
20. Ibid., 164.
21. Boothman., 31.
22. Ibid., 29.

23. Ibid., 31.
24. Ibid.
25. Ibid., 14.
26. Robert Norton, *Communicator Style: Theory, Application, and Measures* (Beverly Hills: Sage Publications, 1983), 106.
27. Boothman, 14.
28. Ibid., 47.
29. Leil Lowndes, *How To Talk To Anyone: 92 Little Tricks for Big Success in Relationships* (New York: Contemporary Books, 2003), 3.
30. Virginia P. Richmond and James C. McCroskey, *Nonverbal Behavior in Interpersonal Relations* (Boston: Pearson, 2004), 65.
31. Boothman, 14.
32. Lowndes, *How To Talk to Anyone*, 15.
33. Ibid.
34. Roger E. Axtell, *Gestures: The Do's and Taboos of Body Language around the World* (New York: John Wilsey and Sons, Inc., 1998), 67.
35. Boothman, 15.
36. Lowndes, 8.
37. Boothman, 15.
38. Ibid., 16.
39. Richmond and McCroskey, 66.
40. Boothman, 16.
41. Axtell, *Gestures*, 122.
42. Ibid., 36.
43. T. Dean Thomlison, *Toward Interpersonal Dialogue* (New York: Longman, 1982), 48.
44. Boothman, 72.
45. Ibid., 72.
46. Ibid., 90.
47. Anderson, *Conversation, Language, and Possibilities*, 144.
48. Ibid., 145.
49. Boothman, 91.
50. Ibid., 90.
51. Anderson, 146.
52. Ibid., 46.
53. Boothman, 92.
54. Ibid.
55. Ibid.
56. Ibid., 103.
57. Purdy and Borisoff, 1.
58. Ibid., 2.
59. Boothman., 103.
60. Anderson, 46.
61. Ibid., 153.

62. Dennis M. Kratz and Abby Robinson Kratz, *Effective Listening Skills* (Chicago: Mirror Press, 1995), 20.
63. Kratz and Kratz, 20.
64. Boothman, 103.
65. Anderson, 154.
66. Leslie A. Baxter and Barbara Montgomery, *Relating: Dialogues and Dialectics* (New York: The Guildford Press, 1996), 238.
67. John Shotter, *Conversational Realities: Constructing Life through Language* (London: Sage Publications, 1993), 39.
68. Kratz and Kratz, 21.
69. Purdy and Borisoff, 49.
70. Ibid.
71. Richard Bandler and John Grinder, as quoted in Nicholas Boothman, *How to Make People Love You in 90 Seconds or Less* (New York: Workman Publishing, 2000), xiv.
72. Nicholas Boothman, *How To Make People Love You in 90 Seconds or Less* (New York: Workman Publishing, 2004), 217.
73. Boothman, *How To Make People Like You*, 115.
74. Ibid., 131.

Chapter Three

Pastoral Conversations with Hospital Patients

THE IMPORTANCE OF GOOD COMMUNICATION SKILLS IN A HEALTH CARE SETTING

In this chapter, we discuss communication skills which can be learned and practiced by pastoral ministers and other caregivers. These skills are intended to build rapport and move conversation, mutually, toward the type of content, clarity, depth, and understanding directly related to a particular service or discipline. These skills may be applied to other caregivers besides pastoral ministers. For example, a social worker may be organizing a discharge plan and summary, or a nurse may be orienting a patient to the hospital room, or a dietician may be educating a patient about a new diabetic diet plan. All of these caregivers can build emotional rapport and relationship with their clients.

The pastoral minister, in giving care to patients, establishes rapport and also wants to gather important information, i.e., the patient's thoughts and feelings about being ill and being hospitalized. For example, the pastoral minister is concerned about the patient's spiritual life and practices, interpersonal relationships, and relationship with God. These are often very personal and private areas of a person's life. Eliciting information could easily be experienced as invasive, especially if the pastoral minister is an unfamiliar person with no prior relationship with the patient.

It is within the scope of the pastoral minister's duties to gather information that helps him to better understand his patients. The pastoral minister should be an incarnational person, recognizing Christ in others and in himself. With a sense of reverence and awe, he should embody the ministry of Christ and the Church. Other hospital caregivers are also free to bring this incarnational belief and dynamic to their encounter with patients according to the extent their professions allow.

Building rapport, which is all about trust, is basic. Establishing rapport is like building a house on rock instead of sand. Good rapport presupposes a patient's confidence in the pastoral minister when there is a substantive prior relationship. When there is minimal or no prior relationship between the pastoral minister and patient, advanced rapport building skills are required. The burden is on the pastoral caregiver to learn and practice these skills so as to build upon or build a new pastoral relationship which can, in turn, enable a patient to communicate more openly while having an abiding sense and assurance that the person in whom he is confiding is caring and trustworthy.

THE SKILLS FOR ESTABLISHING IMMEDIATE RAPPORT WITH THE PATIENT

When the pastoral minister meets with a patient for the first time, there may be hesitancy on the patient's part to trust the pastoral minister's care and competencies. The pastoral minister must not assume the trust of the patient but must start building rapport and have a fairly good idea of what to provide. When the pastoral minister's visit is a follow-up visit, a continuation of rapport building is necessary.

In some situations, as when the pastoral minister is a local pastor visiting a church member, usually some level of rapport has already been established (*rapport by nature*), as discussed in chapter two. However, most encounters between pastoral ministers and patients in health care facilities are first time-meetings. Applying the following rapport skills of a first meeting is necessary in order for the goals of the pastoral visit to be achieved. Most of the skills discussed here have already been discussed in chapter two. These skills are very simple and abounding in common sense. I am intentionally applying them to successful conversation with patients.

ENTERING THE PATIENT'S ROOM

Most encounters between a patient and a pastoral minister take place in the patient's room. The impression the pastoral minister makes within the first few seconds of an encounter matters. If the pastoral minister makes the right impressions, the patient sees the pastor as a friend who is sincere, safe, and trustworthy. Whether the door of the room is closed or open, the pastoral minister needs to get permission before entering the patient's room. In some cases, the pastoral minister may need the permission of the nurse or the permission of the patient's family member.

Under normal conditions, there should always be a response from either the patient or from the nurse or from the family members allowing the pastor to enter. The pastoral minister might inquire from the nurse whether the patient was given some sleep-inducing medicine. If this is the case, the pastor may not wake the patient without the permission of the nurse.

There may be the rare case when the pastoral minister, after knocking on the door, may not receive any response. This may happen when the patient is asleep or unconscious, and there is no nurse or family member in the room. The pastoral minister might gently open the door to learn if anyone is inside the room. If the patient is asleep, the pastoral minister can decide whether to rouse the patient or not. If a patient becomes angry at being aroused, the pastoral minister can apologize and negotiate for a different visiting time.

The Introduction/Greeting

The following skills have also been discussed in chapter two. The intention of presenting them here is not to repeat them but to apply them to meaningful conversation with hospital patients.

After the permission to enter is given, the pastoral minister enters the room and starts with a positive attitude of greeting the patient and introducing himself. It is important for the pastoral minister to wash his hands before having any contact with the patient. The washing of hands avoids spreading germs and is also an expression of caring. While washing, the pastoral minister may speak to the patient or use the time silently to prepare himself.

When meeting the patient, especially for the first time, the pastoral minister has to keep his body language open and seem easy to approach. The pastoral minister opens his heart metaphorically and physically upon meeting the patient. This open body language suggests to the patient that the pastoral minister is friendly, cooperative, and is willing to interact with the patient. This openness creates an opportunity to go further to build more rapport with the patient.

To show a positive attitude to the patient, the pastoral minister has to take the lead in making eye contact with the patient. This involves looking directly into the eyes of the patient. Eye contact can produce a feeling of respect and affection in the person being visited. Looking away from the patient may signal lack of interest, may suggest a lack of warmth, or perhaps be a sign of shyness.

While looking directly into the eyes of the patient, the pastoral minister offers a beaming smile to the patient to indicate happiness at seeing the patient.

This gesture may help the patient to accept the pastor as a friend who has come to identify with him. In order for the patient to see the smile as real or genuine, the pastoral minister must make eye contact before smiling.

The pastoral minister should initiate a verbal greeting. Also, it is better to name the patient in greeting if the pastoral minister knows the patient's name, perhaps by consulting the list of patients. The use of names may have cultural and social implications. In the United States, initial contacts should be a bit formal and first names avoided.

The pastoral minister might greet patients in any of these ways: "Hi, Mr. Smith," or "Hello, Ms. Smith." The pastoral minister should also ask the patient the preferred name. It is the adult patient who gives permission to use a first name or nickname. Whether the pastoral minister knows the name of the patient or not, the pastoral minister should also introduce himself and use his title and names: "Hi, Mr. Smith. My name is Pastor Stewart Jonas."

When ministering to children, the pastoral minister may be a bit careful not to start interacting with a child without the presence or the consent either of the parents or the nurse. In calling the child by name, the pastoral minister may not be as formal as when ministering to adults. The first name of the child may be used.

During the introduction, the pastoral minister leans forward, especially when giving the patient a handshake. This action indicates openness and interest in meeting the patient. It could also be a sign of respect for the patient. The lean can create intimacy between the pastoral minister and the patient.

The pastoral minister might then initiate a handshake if the patient is a man. The pastoral minister should not necessarily initiate a handshake with a female patient. Because some cultures prefer a gentle grip to a firm grip, the pastoral minister should know what is acceptable in the culture where he or she is doing ministry. However, in the hospital environment, a gentle grip is preferable. A firm handshake can be, at times, overpowering and painful, especially if the patient has arthritis or chronic pain in the hands or wrists. Allowing the patient to determine the strength of the grip is suggested.

Synchronizing/Matching

Rapport building does not end at the greeting stage as previously described. The pastor may continue building rapport by synchronizing with the actions of the patient. Synchronizing is simply adjusting behavior to look like that of the patient. It involves matching the patient's mood and effect, voice tone, volume, breathing rate, and body posture, without compromising personal standards and values. Not compromising means that the pastoral minister should not synchronize negative actions or words from the patient. For example, the pastoral minister should not synchronize the racist or profane or angry words used by the patient. Rather, the pastoral minister should synchronize the emotions of the patient. If the patient is in a sad mood, the pastoral minister may also look sad as the patient. Under normal conditions, synchronization makes for more effective rapport and helps to connect the patient and the pastoral minister.

While the pastoral minister is entering the patient's room and introduces himself, it is advisable for the pastoral minister to assess the mood of the patient. Looking at the face of the patient, the pastoral minister may find that the patient looks angry, sad, depressed, content, or perhaps even happy. It is important for the pastor to comment on the mood of the patient for clarity.

Matching the patient's mood can help the patient to accept the pastoral minister's caring gestures. Though the pastoral minister should initiate a smile during the introduction stage, it must be withdrawn if the patient does not smile back. The patient may be in pain and may not be ready to smile. If the pastoral minister keeps smiling while the patient is in a sad mood, the patient is obviously not in sync with the pastoral minister. The pastoral minister may greet a patient with a loud, energetic tone, but if the patient replies slowly in a low tone, the pastor should match and speak slowly in a low tone. Matching the patient's low tone and slow speech does not mean parroting or repeating what the patient is saying. The slow and low tone of the patient could be an indication that the patient is not feeling comfortable. Mismatching or continuing to act happy while the patient is sad can lead to a disconnection after initial rapport has been established.

One day when called to visit a patient in a local hospital, I entered the room and introduced myself by saying, "Hi, Ms. Douglas. My name is Pastor Cajetan. I was passing by and wanted to check on how you were doing." While introducing myself, I had observed that her facial expression and voice tone seemed sad. I commented on this, saying, "Ms. Douglas, it looks as if you're not feeling so happy this morning. I'm sorry if I'm wrong. Help me understand because I'm interested in how you're feeling."

She answered, "Thank you, sir. You're correct. I'm not feeling so good this morning."

"Ms. Douglas, I'm sorry you're not feeling good." Apart from saying sorry to her, I also synchronized and looked sad like she did. She spoke to me in a low tone while I synchronized by responding in a low tone. My actions were empathetic enough to encourage Ms. Douglas to relax a bit and to talk with me as a friend who had come to share her feelings.

One of the major reasons for matching is to build the type of rapport that enables honest sharing between the pastoral minister and the patient. Matching also enables the pastoral minister to develop the type of rapport that can enable him to lead the patient from one emotional state to another—either intentionally and with agreement with the patient or indirectly.

DIALOGICAL CONVERSATION AT BEDSIDE WITH PATIENT

After applying the introductory skills and synchronizing some of the patient's behaviors, enough rapport may be established for a conversation to start. If there is a seat in the room, it is better for a pastoral minister to sit down before a conversation begins. The pastoral minister should politely ask permission to sit.

As mentioned above in my visit with Ms. Douglas, my comment about her mood is a good example of a "rapport-inducing statement,"[1] a comment that reveals how she felt. Her response was an opportunity for me to ask her a conversational question[2] that would encourage her to speak and give me more detailed information about her feelings or to tell her story while I listened. When I heard that she was not feeling well, I responded by asking, "Could you please *tell* me *why* you are not feeling good? I am sorry to ask, if this is private to you. If you do not mind, I would like to know what is going on or what your doctor is saying. Talk to me, Ms. Douglas. I am a good listener." This question and the following comments gave Ms. Douglas the opportunity to talk in detail about her illness while I applied the listening skills. The need to ask conversational questions should not be an opportunity for the pastoral minister to make the whole conversation a questioner-oriented encounter,[3] as if in a law court.

Although asking conversational questions may help a patient to talk in detail about his illness, some pastoral ministers may prefer not to ask questions, but instead use comments that invite responses from patients. Because other caregivers—doctors, nurses, therapists, social workers—ask patients numerous questions about how they feel, the pastoral minister may chose not to follow this pattern. This method of not asking questions is called *pattern interruption*. By not asking questions, the pastoral minister may invite patients to better express themselves. For example, instead of asking, "Ms. Douglas, how are you feeling?" the pastoral minister who does not want to ask questions may say, "Ms. Douglas, I believe that it does help to talk about things. Others think and feel differently. I'm here and I care about you if you would like to share." Both statements invite Ms. Douglas to say how she is feeling. The pastoral minister is, of course, free to use any pattern that best serves his pastoral purpose or to use both.

ACTIVE LISTENING TO THE PATIENT

Active listening involves making attempts to grasp, understand, and feel the emotion that motivates the patient to talk, a listening that takes place at the same time that the pastoral minister responds with appropriate feedback. Active listening also involves absorbing what the patient is saying and applying the skills that would make the patient feel that the pastor is interested in what he or she is saying.[4] In my visit with Ms. Douglas, I asked an open or conversational question that encouraged her to tell me her story. As she talked, I focused my attention on her and nodded my head occasionally to indicate that I was paying attention to what she was saying. I also looked into her eyes to indicate that I was listening.[5] Sometimes, I synchronized her body movement and the movement of her arms. I occasionally made such comments as, "You're right, and I understand what you're saying." These comments encouraged her to talk more.

Recognizing the Patient's Sensory Preferences in the Conversation

Recognizing the sensory preferences or the "favorite sense" of a conversation partner (in getting or giving information), and synchronizing it, contributes to effective rapport. To be able to recognize the favored sense of a conversation partner, the pastoral minister has to listen very attentively. In my conversation with Ms. Douglas, I listened carefully to discover whether she was using visual words (sight) or auditory words (hearing) or kinesthetic words (feeling). Having asked Ms. Douglas to tell me if there was any improvement in her condition, she sighed and said, "I do not *believe* that my condition is improving as fast as I expected. They didn't seem to know just what is wrong with me. I keep having pains in my lower abdomen. I am *frustrated*. I want home soon."

I replied, "Sorry, Ms. Douglas, I do not blame you. When I had a headache last week, I took pain-relieving pills expecting it to go away fast, but it continued and the medicine didn't touch the pain. I was *frustrated* and *unhappy* too. However, I felt better after a day or two."

Ms. Douglas used several kinesthetic words in describing her condition. Her repeated use of feeling terms helped me discover that the favored sense of Ms. Douglas' was primarily kinesthetic. I replied by also using the similar type of words. The point of using the feeling words was to enhance rapport to help Ms. Douglas became more connected to me.

As our discussion went on, I discovered that Ms. Douglas' mood was changing. She did not look as unhappy as she had looked before our conversation began. She seemed cheerful. When she smiled occasionally, I responded to her action with a smile. My interest and responses to her seemed to bring a change. She was no longer expressing her earlier unhappiness and bad feeling. Her attention was more on narrating to me what was happening within her. I observed a positive shift in her mood.

Approach and Comments

Ms. Douglas' situation is a good example of a patient who was ready to talk, but only after some rapport had been established. However, there are situations where the patient may not be ready to talk even after rapport is attempted. Some patients may be unconscious or too weak to talk or may be angry at the Church or at God for whom the pastoral minister represents. If the pastoral minister applies the rapport skills and the patient does not feel like talking, the pastoral minister should not put pressure on the patient.

The approach on Ms. Douglas above is called *identification.* I identified with Ms. Douglas in her painful and frustrating experiences by telling her about my own painful headache. Identification with a patient in this way creates a common ground between the pastoral minister and the patient. When the patient views the pastoral minister as having had similar experiences, this helps the pastoral minister to gain more credibility with the patient. This approach can also encourage the sick person to exercise patience and hope for survival. The pastoral minister may not wish to relate his own experiences to the patient but may instead decide to talk about the experiences of other patients or friends.

A FULL ENCOUNTER WITH A PATIENT: THE CASE OF KEN

I was once asked to go and see a young man in his mid thirties who had indicated to his nurse that he had suffered enough and wanted to end his life. Due to a shooting event that took place when he was twenty-five years old, Ken (not his real name) had been paralyzed from the waist down for about ten years. After spending years in a wheelchair, he was fed up with life. Ken's doctor had just told him that there was no possibility of Ken's walking again. This sad news was so devastating to him that Ken wished for death. Ken even expressed his disappointment with God for not protecting him in the shooting. He had been an altar boy when he was younger and had tried his best to live a good life as a young man. After years of prayers, instead of experiencing healing from God, Ken heard the direct opposite—a prognosis of permanent paralysis.

At the door of his room, I knocked and heard a faint and low voice asking me to come in. When I entered, I looked directly into the eyes of a sad-looking man. I smiled at him, but when he did not return my smile, I withdrew mine. It was then that I suspected that something serious was bothering him. Feeling sad myself, I greeted him in a low tone. "Hi Ken. I'm Pastor Cajetan, a chaplain here. I was passing by and came to express my concern about your being here." He stretched out his hands for a handshake. He said, "Thank you, Pastor, for coming."

"Thanks, Ken, for allowing me to visit with you. You don't look happy this morning. Sorry if I'm wrong, but it looks as if something's really bothering you."

"Yes, Pastor, I feel like taking my own life. I'm tired of this useless life."

"Sorry, Ken. If I may ask, *why* is your life useless? I'm concerned. Talk to me please. I'm ready to listen."

"My life is useless because for the past ten years I've been paralyzed from my waist down. I'm tired of living this way. For a man of my age to depend on others for basically everything I need is not a fun way to live. I *feel* like dying."

"Ken, I *feel* so sad to hear what you're going through. I care about you. As you shared your experiences, there was a pain in my heart, especially when you mentioned your paralysis. It would help me if you could tell me *what* led to your being paralyzed."

"Ten years ago, I was outside my apartment beside my car when I heard gunshots. I was so terrified and didn't know where the gunshots were coming from. I ran out to the street to find out what was happening. I saw the police and a gang of men supposedly selling drugs. The police wanted to arrest them, and when they couldn't, there was a shootout. When I understood what was happening, I tried to run back into my house. A stray bullet hit me in the back. I fell and didn't know what happened to me until the following morning when I found myself in the hospital. I don't really know why God would allow such a thing to happen to me."

"Oh my goodness, I'm very sorry, Ken. That was a terrible and unfortunate experience. Such experience could make anyone ask a lot of questions. Thank you for sharing so much with me. It helps me to understand more your thoughts and feelings at this time. You wondered why God allowed such a thing to happen to you. I would like to hear more about this from you and how you *feel* about God in this condition."

"I am angry at God wherever He is! I still cannot understand why God allowed this to happen to me. This incident has changed my life forever. I have not experienced any improvement for the past ten years now. To die is best. Don't even preach to me or say any prayers in this room. I have prayed for ten years, only to hear from my doctor that I will never walk. Pastor, do not preach or pray for me!

"I have heard you, Ken. I promise to honor your wish, though I hope I am not imposing by sharing a story."

Ken's story and his decision to take his life were so pathetic, I felt so sad. I decided to use a story to help him see his condition differently and possibly to make a wiser decision. This approach is called *leading*. Leading refers to helping a patient to move from one emotional condition to another.

"May I tell you a story?" I asked.

"Go ahead!"

"Many years ago, before the white man came to Africa and brought Christianity, people used to worship the local gods. They used to interpret a lot of things that happened to them according to what they felt about the gods. There was a disease called '*Afor otito*,' which means "swollen stomach." It was a dreaded disease. Anyone with this disease was regarded as an evil human being who had committed an evil act either in this world or in the person's past world, or perhaps his ancestors had done something terrible. Such a disease was seen as punishment from the gods. Our people used to think that illness was a punishment for sin.

"Our people also believed that to avoid attracting the wrath of the gods on the innocent of the village, the sick person would be thrown into the evil forest where it was believed the evil spirits had their dwelling. The person would be rejected by brothers and sisters, parents, friends, and relations and left to die inside the evil forest.

There was a man called Chinwendu (*God Owns Life*) who had lost his wife. He found it very difficult to bear the loss. They had two boys Chika (*God Is Greater*) and Chidi (*There Is God*). Chinwendu's sons were his only consolation. A month after Chinwendu's wife died, he went to the farm to get some yams for the two sons to eat. While at the farm, he heard gun shots in his village. He was very afraid and ran back to learn what was happening."

I noticed a little excitement in Ken as he listened to me, nodding his head and eager to hear more. Because Ken was listening with interest, I continued.

"On reaching the village, Chinwendu saw that it was deserted. He got to his house and didn't see his two sons. He started to search for them only to be told that the village had been attacked by slave-raiders. They had guns to raid villages and to capture people for slavery. By evening of that day, it was discovered that his two sons were among those captured and taken to the slave ship, and there was no hope of seeing them again. It was too much for Chinwendu to bear. This was only a short time after losing his wife. He refused to be consoled. The remaining of the village people gathered every day to console him, but he did not see the need to keep on living.

"One night he made up his mind to take his own life. He had a rope to hang himself. He considered the best place to commit suicide so that people would not know what was happening and try to rescue him. He quietly took his rope and went into the evil forest in the dead of the night. He climbed an Iroko tree and tied the rope around one of the branches. Just as he was about to tie the rope to hang himself, he heard someone calling from the foot of the tree, 'Hey, Chinwendu, if you want to hang yourself, make sure you tie the rope very well so that you don't fall off and hit my swollen stomach and kill me because I am not yet ready to die.'

Chinwendu shouted, 'Who is there?'

'It is me Wereuwakodi (*Take the World as It Is*). Please be careful not to wound me.'

Hearing a voice from the foot of the Iroko tree at that time of the night, Chinwendu was terrified. He immediately removed the rope from his neck and looked down and saw a man with a swollen stomach who had been thrown away by relations to die because of the disease he had."

There was an outburst of laughter by Ken. I laughed as well. I noticed a change in his mood and he sounded more excited. I continued, "Chinwendu hurriedly climbed down the Iroko tree, threw away the rope, and ran away saying, 'Oh my God! Here is a man who has been abandoned to die and he does not want to die, and here I am ready to take my life.'

Chinwendu ran home, and from that day, he accepted life as it came and never again tried to take his life."

Ken burst into laughter again and asked, "Are you sure this happened?"

I laughed along with him and replied, "Yeah, we were told that it happened. It is one of those folk stories told among the Igbos of Eastern Nigeria. There are different versions of it, but it's the same lesson. My uncle told us that it was our great grandfather who told our grandfather the story and our grandfather told him the story, and he handed it down to us when we were still small."

"That is a great story. So what are you trying to tell me? Does it mean that no matter the condition of things, no person should think of killing himself?"

"You have said so, Ken."

"It sounds like something you would see in a movie. However, thank you for telling me the story. I know that it is not right for me to take my life, but there are certain circumstances where ending life seems like the best thing."

"I understand you, Ken. I do not blame you for feeling like ending it. At the same time, I am happy that you listened to my story. I hope you will think about it."

"Well, thank you for telling me the story. I got the meaning. I will think about it."

"Thanks, Ken, for listening. Let me ask you this last question. Is there anyone who loves you so much and you love so much who will be deeply devastated if something else were to happen to you?"

"Yes."

"Who is the person?"

"My mother is the person."

"Tell me about her."

"She was here shortly before you came in. You would have seen her if you had come a bit earlier. She is a sweet mother, and the best mother I can have in this world. She loves me so much and I love her so much. She is my only source of strength."

"Ken, I am happy you have someone who loves you. I am sure you do not want to break her heart. Think about her and think about the story. Let me know if there is any way I can be of help. I will leave you to have some rest now. Once more, thanks for listening to me. I hope to see you soon."

"Thanks a lot, Pastor. Bye."

SHORT ANALYSIS OF THE ENCOUNTER WITH KEN

This encounter with Ken was therapeutic and grace-filled for both of us. We both had stories to tell and needed others to listen to us, value, and appreciate what we had to say. There were sadness and joy in both of our lives. We could talk of happier times and then of significant changes. At the end of our encounter, we both felt differently. We were both at peace with our lives. We had things to think about.

As mentioned earlier, this approach was a good example of what Judith Acosta and Judith Simon Prager call *leading*.[6] By telling Ken my own story, I was able to *lead* him out from his depressed feeling and the thought of taking his life to a more positive feeling of accepting life as it comes. My story also interrupted his cycle of depressive thinking and in this sense could be called a *pattern interruption*.

Recommendations

Under ordinary conditions, the pastoral minister would have prayed with the patient during the visit. I certainly would have liked to pray with Ken, but I remembered that he had said that he wished that I should not.

The approach I used in Ken's case is different from that of Ms. Douglas. After listening to Ken, I told him a folk story, which acted as a metaphor, but, more importantly, as a therapy not only to engage his imagination, but to consider his very life more clearly and seriously. The story of Ken could be viewed and heard through the filter of *parallel process* which a person hears and uses unconsciously as his own self-portrait. From personal experiences, I have noticed that sometimes I tell my audience other peoples' stories without being conscious that I am using such stories to reveal myself.

Documentation of Patient's Story and Ethical Implications

After meeting with the patient, it is helpful for the pastoral minister to reflect on the visit briefly and then document the visit, especially if it is required by the healthcare facility. It is neither proper nor advisable for the pastoral minister to record what the patient is saying about his illness and feelings in his or her presence. If the pastoral minister records or writes down the story while listening, it could lead to suspicion and could make a patient less open or less expressive.

While documenting the patient's story, the real name of the patient should not be used. Documenting the exact name of the patient and using it in public without permission could constitute a serious violation of the privacy policy of the health facility. It could also constitute a violation of HIPAA (Health Insurance Portability and Accountability Act) rules, which provide federal protection for private health information in the hands of health facilities and provides some rights for patients to assure the privacy of their health information.[7]

In the next chapter, we shall discuss the movement of patients' stories and experiences from the bedside to the pulpit. It is one thing for the pastoral minister to gather valuable information from patients; it is another thing for the pastoral minister to know how to use such stories in the preparation and delivery of a sermon.

NOTES

1. Nicholas Boothman, *How To Make People Like You in 90 Seconds or Less* (New York: Workman Publishing, 2000), 91.
2. Harlene Anderson, *Conversation, Language, and Possibilities: A Postmodern Approach to Therapy* (New York: BasicBooks, 1997), 145.
3. Michael Purdy and Deborah Borisoff, eds., *Listening in Everyday Life, Intra/ Interpersonal Listening* (New York: University of America, 1997), 49.
4. Boothman., 103.
5. Dennis M. Kratz and Abby Robinson Kratz, *Effective Listening Skills* (Chicago: Mirror Press, 1995), 21.

6. Judith Acosta and Judith Simon Prager, *The Worst Is Over: Verbal First Aid To Calm, Relieve Pain, Promote Healing and Save Lives* (San Diego, California: Jodere, 2001), 73.

7. US Department of Health and Human Services, "Health Information Privacy," available at www.hhs.gov/ocr/privacy/hipaa/understanding/index.html.

Chapter Four

From Patient's Story to Homily

The encounters between the pastoral minister and the sick do not end merely with listening to their stories. Moving their stories from bedside to pulpit involves a hermeneutical process. We shall therefore examine the hermeneutical process involved in the interaction of human stories (patients') and divine stories (God's) to give birth to a homily that can address the problems of the sick. We shall also refer to sample homilies which are presented in the appendix.

THE ROLE OF STORY IN PREACHING PROCLAMATION

The use of stories to pass on messages from one generation to another is as old as the human race. Stories, good stories, capture the attention of the listeners and engage their curiosity and imagination while opening a doorway to their other-than-conscious minds. Storytelling can be useful to convey knowledge and information, to stimulate creative thinking and reflection, and to subtly and indirectly introduce therapeutic messages. William Nichols observes that the use of stories to relay important messages has been applied frequently and has always yielded remarkable results.[1] According to Ronald J. Allen, "Stories offer a framework of meaning within which to understand persons, relationships, events, actions."[2]

In the Old and New Testaments, stories and shared personal experiences were commonly used to convey divine truths. The story of Job is a good example of a sick person's story, and religious teachers have used this story for many generations to communicate a divine truth about where God is found in human suffering and about how human beings react to their suffering conditions. Sometimes it is difficult to understand why people suffer. When people feel that they do not deserve their suffering conditions, they ask such questions as: Why me? What have I done to deserve this illness? Why has God allowed me to suffer?

Although asking the above questions seems natural, there may not be satisfactory answers. Nevertheless, religious teachers have used Job's story and other stories to communicate that no matter how difficult it is to understand why bad things happen, God does not abandon his people. The suffering receive abundant blessings from God. The blessings of being faithful to God in hard times may be realized in this life or in the life to come.

In the gospels, Jesus also used many stories in addressing his listeners. Nichols sees Jesus as a master storyteller who used stories that carried the burden of the message he wanted to deliver.[3] Jesus got to the heart of his hearers by using many parables, common images, and familiar language that attracted them to listen and understand his message, even when the message was not easily understood and needed some explanation. Luke's Good Samaritan story is an example of a parable used by Jesus to teach his audience the divine truth about the love and hospitality that should be accorded a stranger or a sick person who needs help (Luke 10:30-37).

Contemporary preachers have also realized the effectiveness of using stories and past experiences in preaching to their audiences. Allen acknowledges that stories, images and experiences can be used as effective illustrations that can make the homily more lively and easy to understand, especially when there are abstract theological assertions.[4] Sickness may alienate the sick from their communities, especially when communities do not value and reach out to their sick members. Therefore, when the stories of the sick are incorporated into preaching events, the homilist can reconnect and strengthen the connection between the sick and those who are well. The pastoral minister can also make it known to the members of the community that when one member suffers, all suffer. At the very least, the pastoral minister can remind those who are well of the presence and value of the sick.

By attentively listening to the stories of the sick, other members of the community may identify some "common ground" in their own stories.[5] The stories of the sick become a common ground experience when members of the community find similarities between their own stories and those of the sick, of things they have already experienced, are currently experiencing, or are likely to experience. For example, one hospital worker expressed her appreciation with Homily One. According to her, this homily helped her to understand better what it means when we say that God suffers with us and does not abandon us to suffer alone. When patients' stories are used in homilies, as demonstrated in the appendix, the healthy are encouraged to prepare for a possible challenge of faith through illness. Such stories may act as consolation or encouragement to "God-fearing sufferers."[6]

THE SICK AS SACRAMENT TO THE COMMUNITY

The experiences of the sick contained in their stories are a sacrament through which the Christian community can receive grace. Through sharing the experiences of the sick, especially in liturgical celebrations, the community comes to a better understanding of God's place in the world. The sick person's stories and experiences could act as "evidential experiences"[7] to back up the point about God's grace and love for the sick. An example of an evidential experience is presented in Homily Two.

The encounter between the pastoral minister and the sick is itself a sacrament or a source of grace for the sick, for the pastoral minister, and for the community. This sacramental encounter can be seen in the image of Jesus accompanying his confused, disappointed, and depressed disciples walking from Jerusalem to Emmaus. The disciples received grace through word and sacrament and saw meaning in their depressed condition. In their encounter with Jesus, they received not only hope and grace, they also shared their hope and grace with the Christian community in Jerusalem.

The preacher encounters the sick, listens to their stories, and shares them with the Christian community. These stories become creative elements of our liturgical celebrations and contain within them the reality that they communicate. Just as Christ is present in the word and in the common elements of bread and wine, Christ is present in the common ground stories of the sick. David N. Power states that the word of God ensures eschatological hope, especially in a sacramental encounter. The sick person receives this word in faith, embraces and owns it and becomes, in turn, a sacrament of meaning for the community.[8] For example, after the liturgical celebration in which Homily One was preached, a patient expressed her appreciation of the homily. She indicated that she felt God's love and presence more in her life.

Joye Gros sees the whole act of bringing forth our life experiences, including those of the sick, for reflection as engaging in a deep act of faith.[9] In other words, our faith or the faith of the community is enriched and strengthened when members share their stories with one another.

THE PREACHER AS A THEOLOGICAL REFLECTOR

Moving the patient's stories and experiences from bedside to homiletic proclamation involves a hermeneutical process in which the preacher plays the role of a theological reflector. In the words of Patricia O' Connell Killen and John De Beer, "Theological reflection nurtures growth in faith by bringing life experiences into conversation with the wisdom of the Christian heritage."[10] The pastoral minister as theological reflector must be mature in faith, able to pay attention to the experiences of the sick, and able to inquire about the meaning of these experiences in accordance with their religious heritage.[11]

Experience is what happens to us. Our experiences may spur us to ask questions and invite us to reflect.[12] The sick have experiences that are capable of evoking feelings, thoughts, attitudes, hopes and even despair. The sick are challenged to share their stories honestly. Sharing stories is easier for some than others. While the troubling conditions of the sick may make them ask questions, the sick may not have time and space to reflect well theologically on what is happening to them in their relationships to God, to themselves, to others, and to the world. The pastoral minister can help facilitate this process of reflection with the sick person by listening and helping him to reflect. According to Robert L. Kinast, "The standard technique for representing one's experience is to narrate it, orally or in writing, and usually to people who are prepared to reflect upon it theologically."[13] The hermeneutical process begins when the pastoral minister listens to the experiences of the sick, reflects on them, interprets and applies them to a Christian belief system for better understanding or meaning, and shares this theological reflection with the worshipping community.

The following example shows the beginning of theological reflection. Pat (not her real name) entered the hospital in severe emotional, physical, and spiritual distress. Due to significant health problems, Pat worried that she was losing her trust and faith in God, whom she believed with all her heart, would never give her more than she could bear. The pastoral minister provided Pat ample opportunity to share her story and her feelings without interruption. Sensing her frustration and noting her fears, the pastoral minister asked permission to share a personal reflection. When Pat agreed, the pastoral minister responded that Pat reminded him of Jesus in that she did not deserve this cross, yet carried it though overwhelmed at times. The pastoral minister reflected that Jesus also had stumbled several times under the weight of the cross, but Jesus had help from Simon of Cyrene who carried the cross for a period of time. The pastoral minister suggested that Pat could let someone else shoulder her cross for awhile as well.

After the pastoral minister had finished this theological reflection, Pat expressed that she had never thought of it that way. Pat's statement indicated that the pastoral minister had helped her to begin the process of theological reflection. Later, the pastoral minister might continue this process by moving the patient's experiences from the bedside to the pulpit. In the homily, patients, as well as those in the congregation hearing the story, need to continue the process of reflection even after the liturgical celebration. By the end of this theological reflection process, the pastoral minister should be able to help the sick understand a new meaning to their conditions in accordance with their faith.

When the pastoral minister does theological reflection well, it can enhance healing, as well as encourage understanding and support from the community. Edward O. de Bary suggests that when theological reflection takes place, health is improved because a healthy climate is established. A healthy climate brings about honesty, support, openness, and charity in a community that cares and supports its members.[14]

BEDSIDE ENCOUNTER AND ITS EFFECTS ON THE PASTORAL MINISTER

The homiletic process of using the patient's story in preaching starts at the bedside when the pastoral minister listens to the stories and experiences of the sick person. As the pastoral minister listens attentively, he can find himself empathetically in the shoes of the patient. As David Hogue observes, "Imaginatively participating in a story we are hearing is a consequence of our capacity for empathy."[15] Carrie Doehring also observes that walking in the sick person's shoes or seeing the world from his or her perspective means not only feeling with the sick but also being able to preach from this experience and from the heart.[16] When a pastoral minister preaches from a practical experience, the preaching is more persuasive and effective because it is from the heart. Preaching that is based on personal or practical common ground experience is more effective than preaching based on the prepared homilies or commentaries of others.

Through attentive listening, the preacher can become aware of significant issues in the life of the sick person, and then find ways to address these issues in preaching. "Listening to stories can give us a deeper sense of the meaning that people have made in their lives. The events they include, the ones they omit, and the inevitable embellishments and discounts they make can help us appreciate how the world is constructed for persons who seek our care."[17] The more attentively and accurately the minister listens, the more accurate and focused is the assessment and response, and the minister is less likely to impose his or her own issues, values, and perspectives.

For example, I listened to the story of a sixty-five-year old patient, Mr. Jackson (not his real name), whose greatest disappointment and regret was that his illness and age had created such limitations that he could no longer be active in managing his business effectively. When I entered Mr. Jackson's room and greeted him, he looked at me and asked, "Are you a football player? You look very strong, the way I used to look when I was in my twenties and thirties." In my further discussion with Mr. Jackson, I learned that he used to work three jobs as a young man. Through his hard work, he was able to establish his own business. His company was flourishing before he had the stroke which made it impossible for him to move about and oversee his business. Unfortunately, when his son took over, the son was not able to manage the company effectively. Mr. Jackson lamented, "Regrettably, everything seems to be crumbling in my life. It pains me to hell."

When I first listened to Mr. Jackson, I immediately connected with him because of some similarities in his story and in mine, suggesting identification between the patient and this pastoral minister. I could understand his concerns and what he held important. For example, he and I both valued hard work. When Mr. Jackson commended me as a strong-looking man, I became aware of my own limitations. His story made me realize how limited persons can become due to illness and age. The way I played soccer when I was in my twenties is no longer how I play it now. I see myself becoming limited due to age.

I had to listen on several levels and with all of my senses, with my heart, mind, and imagination. Listening to Mr. Jackson, I later reflected on his story and mine to discover deeper meanings that made me more conscious of my own emotions of which I had been unaware. This process of reflection and unconscious discovery of deeper meaning and common ground in the story of the pastoral minister and that of the patient is called *parallel process*. Gerald Egan suggests that the pastoral minister not only listens to the words of others, but he also listens to the message buried in the words or encoded in the cues that surround the words.[18] Stories truly reveal much about the teller and not only create a feeling of empathy for the listener but also help the listener to reflect on some personal realities.

In preaching, the pastoral minister is professionally obliged to use this *parallel process* both to better understand and appreciate other-than-conscious connections or disconnections with the patient and his story. Parallel process should monitor any subsequent sermons, so that they are of God and for the people of God and not personal messages and revelations.

TYPES OF STORIES AS GIFTS TO PREACHING

When individuals are subjected to physical or mental pain due to illness or other sources of suffering, they react against their experiences differently and in a variety of ways. Some patients may want to talk or express their feelings by telling stories, while some may not want to talk. Some may talk but may not be talking coherently, especially some patients in psychiatric units. Not all stories or reactions to illnesses may be good resource materials for preaching. However, by applying the skills discussed in chapter three, the preacher listens attentively for the following gifts from the patient's stories and experiences.

LISTENING FOR THE GIFTS OF QUESTION AND CHALLENGE

When listening to the stories of the sick, the pastoral minister occasionally hears patients ask challenging questions. In order to understand their depressing conditions and the reasons for their suffering, some patients may demand answers of God. Wayne E. Oates asserts, "They may even quite legitimately rail out against God for his mistreatment of them."[19] Joyce Travelbee posits that these questions indicate the patients' non-acceptance of illness and suffering and their desire to get well or be healed.[20] Asking questions to understand their suffering conditions may also show the extent to which illness has challenged their faith and may reveal the problems of fear and impatience connected to illness. Though it may seem negative to ask God questions, these questions can provide insights for the pastoral minister to reflect and to address some problems such as fear, impatience, and challenge to faith.

For example, by listening to Ken's story of his pain and paralysis, the preacher understood that Ken felt unjustly treated by God and questioned his suffering. Ken's questions came out of fear and the desperate desire to get well. His questions were similar to those of Job in the Scriptures. Hearing such questions and observing the extent to which the faith of the patient is challenged, the pastoral minister should take note because many other patients may be asking similar questions and may be challenged in similar ways. Such questions and challenges act as good resource materials to be used in later homilies. Ken's story, a suitable example of the gifts of question and challenge, is presented in Homily One.

LISTENING FOR THE GIFTS OF BLAME AND DESPAIR

Sometimes, while narrating their experiences, the pastoral minister may hear patients blame themselves for their illnesses. A person who develops lung cancer after repeated warnings by his physician to stop heavy smoking may blame himself for acting against medical advice and for contributing to his illness and suffering.[21] This kind of response was evident in the story of Joey who blamed himself for his paralysis and for causing the death of his two friends because Joey had driven while under the influence of alcohol.

There are some people who blame God for not protecting them when they suffer in an accident. Frequently, there is anger especially when the individual did not cause the accident. A pastoral minister may also hear some patients refer to their illnesses as "punishments" from God—either for going against their religious teachings or for living careless lifestyles. Many HIV patients blame themselves or are blamed by others for being responsible for their suffering.

Patients who blame themselves for causing their illnesses and sufferings sometimes talk with despair as if they have lost the hope of being forgiven by God. Though pastoral ministers may want to help such patients find relief and forgiveness, they should allow such patients sufficient time to talk about their guilt, shame, blame, and responsibility. However, it is important for the pastoral minister to notice such signs of despair. These signs can provide rich resource materials for preaching. While the gospel should provide a message of hope for such patients, the pastoral minister should include a strong message of hope in the homily.

LISTENING FOR THE GIFTS OF WITNESS, ACCEPTANCE, AND HOPE

While listening to patients, the pastoral minister should note those who, through their stories, display acceptance of their suffering conditions as a way of expressing their faith or bearing witness to their religious belief. Such expressions of faith while undergoing suffering provide good resource material that can be used for preaching. These patients have not given up hope for healing and for life even when their illnesses may be terminal. In the words of Travelbee, "Their acceptance is based on a realization of the human condition combined with a profound belief in the tenets of their creed. In order to demonstrate this type of acceptance, an individual must have firmly believed, as well as followed his religious convictions."[22]

Such patients have come to terms with illness and have resigned their fate to whatever God allows. They also demonstrate hope of healing, even when their illnesses are critical or terminal. They believe that the reward of eternal life awaits them. Coming to terms with illnesses does not mean that such patients do not express fear and pain. As Travelbee puts it, "This is not to say that such a person never wavers, is never anxious, or never needs reassurance or encouragement. It does mean, however, that such a person is able to bear the weight of these sufferings over a long period of time with patience and a type of serene resignation."[23]

In my hospital ministry, I was surprised at an encounter with Jane, a fifty-year-old cancer patient. She expressed that she was in terrible pain. It was not clear if she was going to survive her current hospitalization. Jane related how terrible she was feeling and I asked her how she felt about God in her illness. She told me that if not for God, her illness could have been worse. She also told me that she had handed herself and her sufferings over to God and was ready for whatever would come. I was amazed by her responses. I had expected her to talk angrily and to lash out at God for her incurable illness. Jane was definitely ready for death and had hope of a new life in God. Jane's expression of faith in the midst of illness is presented in Homily Two.

SELECTION OF TEXT FROM THE CHURCH LECTIONARY OR AS CHOSEN BY THE PREACHER

Hospital preaching may be part of formal Sunday worship or daily liturgical worship or informal gatherings to pray and to share God's word in a way that addresses the conditions of the sick. In these ways, the Scripture is read or quoted and the Word of God is reflected upon and shared among the sick and the healthy. The pastoral minister can choose the text directly from the Bible or follow the selections from the lectionary. William Skudlarek insists that Scripture is the center or core of preaching.[24] Consequently, either way is acceptable.

SELECTION FROM THE BIBLE

Selection from the Bible involves the free choice of a pastoral minister to select a preaching text directly from the Scriptures. One advantage of this free choice of a Biblical text is that it gives the pastoral minister the opportunity to select passages providing a pastoral response or an answer to human conditions or current pressing problems of the sick. This kind of preaching addresses the people here and now and in a way that can touch their lives. Skudlarek calls it "the life-situation approach to preaching."[25]

A disadvantage of choosing directly from the Bible is that it puts the congregation at the mercy of whatever the preacher wishes to preach about. Free choice may also contribute to the preacher frequently return to passages easily preached.[26] By using favorite passages, the preacher gives some problems or issues more attention than others.

Another disadvantage of free choice of a biblical text is that it seems to make the audience the source of the message instead of the receiver of the message. The Bible may seem a mere answer book to problems that may not have existed when the Scriptures were written.[27] Allen observes that in pleasing the congregation or in making them hear what they would like to hear, there may be the tendency of the pastoral minister to avoid some texts that may challenge the hearers to certain demands of the gospel.[28]

LECTIONARY PREACHING

Lectionary preaching involves preaching according to a formal collection of readings from the Scriptures arranged and intended for proclamation either in daily or Sunday liturgical celebrations. This arrangement has an advantage. It helps the pastoral minister and the faithful to prepare ahead of time for the liturgy and the sharing of the word.[29]

Skudlarek suggests that the clergy and the laity gather before the celebration and discuss the readings and pray over them. In health facilities where there are liturgical committees, chaplains and interested health workers may discuss the readings and find ways to apply them to the health care context. In one of the parishes where I lived, we had liturgical committees that gathered once a week to discuss the readings and prepare the liturgy beforehand. The liturgical committee helped to apply the readings to current happenings in the community. If this collaborative handling of the liturgy is applied in health facilities, it may help make the liturgy a shared effort by the pastoral ministers or chaplains, health workers, and perhaps even the sick who may have been resourceful by sharing their stories. As the lectionary is designed to proclaim the paschal mystery of Christ, hospital preaching easily focuses on Christ's teaching on suffering, illness, death, life, hope, resurrection, and other related issues.[30]

However, preaching to the sick from the lectionary has its own problems. Skudlarek observes that the readings have been chosen for specific days without much reference to the needs or the interests of the faithful and the preacher. The readings sometimes are connected to feasts and celebrations that may not be very relevant to the sick.[31] The readings may not address the present pressing problems of the people including the sick. Because of the abstract nature of some of the lectionary readings, the preacher may be at a loss for a message.

ABSTRACT LECTIONARY TEXTS AND PREACHING TO THE SICK

What happens when the readings or the texts assigned to a particular day are so abstract that the pastoral minister finds them very difficult to connect to the needs of the sick? Is liturgical preaching meant only to solve people's problems? Clearly, not. While it is true that liturgical preaching is more effective when it addresses the needs or contemporary problems of the congregation, liturgical preaching is not limited to these needs. Liturgical preaching to the sick should be first and foremost a proclamation of the Word of God. Most readings for the liturgical celebration are Christ-centered. Preaching to the sick should be presented in such a way that the sick see their present conditions in the light of the life, teachings, death, and resurrection of Christ. Daniel Harris asserts that "the Eucharistic homily is a special time when the people of God gather for a unique experience of encountering God in the living word."[32]

When the pastoral minister must address a particular problem and the texts assigned by the lectionary for that particular day make it very difficult for the preacher, Skudlarek has this advice to give:

> In any event, if the situation is of such importance that you must speak to it directly, and if the pericopes assigned for that particular day do not provide you with an appropriate word, no matter how diligently you have sought to hear one there, then by all means choose readings that do enable you to preach the word of the Lord. But do not (repeat, do not) read the lessons from the lectionary and then ignore them completely in your preaching. To do so is a clear, indeed eloquent, way of informing the congregation that the liturgy is something we do because we have to, but that it really doesn't have anything to do with life.[33]

In other words, if the pastoral minister has a pressing issue he desperately needs to address and the readings of the day do not have any connection to the issue, he can put the lectionary readings aside and choose a more suitable reading. As already indicated, it is only in rare situations when the preacher may experience this problem. Directly or indirectly, most readings have words for the sick in their situations. Having been involved in preaching to the sick for a number of years, I have found few instances when I needed to substitute more suitable readings. Moreover, because the hospital community embraces the sick as well as those who serve them, the pastoral minister can also consider the pastoral needs of the hospital staff, families, and friends of the sick.

A THREE-WAY HERMENEUTICS

Preaching to the sick in a health facility involves a three-way hermeneutics or interpretation of the patient's community, the patient's story, and God's own story (Biblical text). The major aim of carrying out this three-way interpretation is to meet the needs of the sick, who in their lived-experiences are struggling with finding new meaning. According to Scott Kevin Davis:

> Exploring meaning is a search for congruity and correlation of their personal story with communal story and a transcendent story. The exploration for and expression of meaning and understanding is the process of hermeneutics. Hermeneutics is the process whereby persons in storied conversation recover old meanings and discover new understanding of experience while critically assessing current interpretations held by both individual and community. . . . Through the hermeneutic process, persons and communities mediate the world in which they live and interact. Through hermeneutics, persons and communities make and remake their understandings of their storied place as individuals and communities. Through hermeneutics, storied life experiences are connected, interpreted, explained, and understood within a larger narrative context.[34]

INTERPRETING THE COMMUNITY OF THE SICK

The hospital community is made up of the sick, health workers, families, relations, and friends of the sick. Members of the hospital community, especially the sick and often their relatives, are persons who have suffered much from problems such as: pain, guilt, shame, punishment, anger, depression, isolation, abandonment, addiction, grief, and loss.

The preacher must study the congregation to be able to structure a homily in context. In *Preaching as Local Theology of Folk Art*, Leonora Tubbs Tisdale describes contextual preaching as involving a strong, growing understanding of the congregation and its cultures. The goal of preparing a homily and delivering it in context is to make the art of preaching more suitable, adaptive, and transformative to the listeners.[35] Preaching to a health care community demands the preacher be well acquainted with the community.

Killen and De Beer, recommend that the preacher consider attitudes, opinions, beliefs, and convictions of the members of the community. The pastoral minister should bear in mind that the behavior of the sick person may be very different from that of the healthy. Due to their conditions, the sick may be very emotional. The language the preacher uses in his homily must be carefully chosen so as not to say anything that could make them react negatively to their conditions. For example, the preacher should not speak as if he is judgmental about what caused their illness. The preacher should use words that can help make them feel accepted, loved, cared for, and offer words that can provide hope.

Preaching to a hospital community also demands that the preacher should know the appropriate message and length of message for the congregation and be attentive to the message without spending too much time in delivery. For a variety of practical reasons, most daily liturgies or masses in hospital settings are about thirty minutes or less. The length of time for liturgies varies for pastoral reasons. Liturgies are usually shortened because of the weakened condition of patients and the frequent, urgent demands placed on hospital personnel.

The pastoral minister cannot afford to mention real names of patients or descriptions of patients that would identify them or reveal the health information of any patient. Revealing such information constitutes a serious violation of the Health Insurance Portability and Accountability Act (HIPAA) rules and professional healthcare ethics.

INTERPRETING THE BIBLICAL TEXT

When interpreting the Biblical text for preaching within a public liturgy, the pastoral minister needs to recognize that those who are sick must encounter new ways of understanding in light of the gospel message. It is the responsibility of the pastoral minister to help the congregation or the hospital community to interpret the meaning of the text as it applies to their present condition in accordance with their tradition. As Allen states, "The preacher helps the Christian community interpret the divine character, the situation of the world, God's relationship to it, and how to respond in ways that are consistent with the gospel."[36]

When preparing to preach, the pastoral minister considers the following questions: What is the text saying? What is the central theme of the text? What problem or problems does the central theme resolve or try to address? The pastoral minister prepares a homily that is sensitive to the concerns of the sick (fear, pain, abandonment, anger, depression, etc). Eugene Lowry proposes this question: "What kerygmatic theme implied in the text provides the clue for resolution?"[37] The resolution of the problems of the sick does not necessarily mean answering all their questions but rather using the kerygmatic message to help them to a better understanding of their situation. A kerygmatic theme refers to a doctrinal truth, revealed as the good news of God's saving action in Christ.[38] Examples of kerygmatic or doctrinal themes include the resurrection, love, forgiveness, Trinity, and so on. If the text indicates a doctrinal theme, the pastoral minister prepares a sermon based on these or similar themes, with special concern for the problems of the sick which these themes seem to address.[39] For example, if a pastoral minister is thinking of preparing a sermon on the resurrection, the primary question is "What problem does the resurrection solve?" With any theme the preacher must focus on a message of hope for the sick.

Eugene Lowry believes that the above process is important, especially for those preachers whose texts are from the lectionary and whose sermons have much to do with biblical interpretation.[40] However, he argues that it is not enough to consider the question of *what* the text is saying, but also to consider *why* the text is saying what it says.[41] In most cases the question of *why* helps the pastoral minister in determining the form the homily should take. Lowry asserts, "Every explicit theme presumes an implicit problem; every explicit problem presumes an implicit theme."[42] It is difficult for a pastoral minister to construct a sermon if the above assertion does not apply.

INTERPRETING AND SELECTING THE APPROPRIATE STORY

To find new meaning in order to cope, the sick consciously or unconsciously tell stories about their lives and what is happening in their lives. Liturgical preaching is, therefore, an opportunity for the preacher to interpret the patient's story, know the problems to be addressed, and connect them to the gospel narratives. For example, Ken's story in chapter three was the story of a frustrated and angry man. It is a good example of extended suffering. His suffering for many years combined with the sad news from his doctor had made him lose interest in continuing with this life. He was also disappointed with God whom he felt should have protected him. Ken's story raises a lot of questions. Why is it that sometimes, God allows suffering? An interpretation of Ken's story then reveals the problems of depression, disappointment, despair, anger, sadness, and limitation. After interpreting the story, the pastoral minister should know if the story can be used as resource material for preaching.

In selecting the appropriate story to proclaim the gospel, the preacher should consider the following:

1) How does the story raise questions and challenge faith? Ken's story, for instance, (Homily One) was a gift of question and challenge to faith.
2) Does the story raise the problems of blame and despair? Joey's story in chapter one, presents these problems as gifts.
3) Does the story indicate a witness to the gospel? Does it reveal acceptance of a suffering condition or can it be seen as a model of Christian life? The story of Jane in Homily Two demonstrates a gift of witness, acceptance, and hope. In plotting the homily, the pastoral minister should be able to know which story is most appropriate for proclaiming the gospel.

RITUALIZATION OF THE PATIENT'S STORY: LINKING GOD'S STORY WITH THE HUMAN STORY

Herbert Anderson and Edward Foley recommend that after listening to the story of the patient, the preacher must ritualize or connect the patient's story to God's own story.[43] The importance of linking God's story and the human story is to help patients reconstruct their lives and see their story as part of God's story.

When I visited hospital patients who had watched the celebration of Mass on closed-circuit television, they would indicate that they felt I spoke directly to them. They did not know that it was the information I had gleaned from listening to previous patients which had prepared me to preach to others. Some of the patients seemed to have applied the homilies personally to themselves and so found their spiritual needs met. The homilies had some transforming effect on them.[44] Anderson and Foley assert, "The potential for a personally and communally transformative encounter is significantly magnified when the divine and the human intersect in our storytelling and ritualizing."[45] The sick see the presence of God in their stories or find their place in the divine narrative. The Biblical narratives have a lot to tell about pain, loss, anger, disappointment, loneliness, abandonment, guilt, shame, and other problems of life. Their expressions of happiness after listening to such homilies suggest that the sick are transformed when they understand their personal stories as a part of a larger transcendent narrative.

PLOTTING THE HOMILY

After interpreting the Biblical texts along with the patient's story, the pastoral minister should have some important information that could be used in plotting the homily. For example, the Biblical text may reveal a central theme or message, while the patient's story may reveal a felt need or an issue that needs to be addressed. What preoccupies the mind of the pastoral minister after interpreting the text and the patient's story? Is it a central Biblical message or is it a felt need or problem? As Lowry indicates, whichever it is, the pastoral minister should look for the opposite.[46]

On plotting the homily, Lowry advocates forming and shaping a sermon by an interaction of problem and theme. In other words, it will involve an interaction between the patient's story and God's story. "When a theme of a proposed sermon is thrown against a problem, a sermon idea may be born. When a problem is pushed against the gospel, the interaction may give birth to a sermon."[47] For Lowry, a preacher who concentrates his sermon on the central message or theme will produce a sermon that sounds like a lecture, which may be strong in content but weak in engaging the audience.[48] On the other hand, Lowry believes that if a preacher concentrates his sermon on a felt need, he will be able to establish a quick contact or rapport with the congregation, but his sermon will be weak in content.

Lowry uses the imagery of *itch* and *scratch* to describe the relationship between the felt need and the message. A sermon should involve both an *itch* and a *scratch*. A homily comes into being when the problematic *itch* intersects the solutional *scratch*.[49] An elementary example of this would connect the patient's fear of death and dying with a Scriptural response about resurrection and new life.

THE PREACHING TEXT: AN EXCITING MESSAGE OF HOPE

The goal of the pastoral minister is to present a message of hope that can transform the lives of the sick. The homily should be plotted and presented as a message of hope to the sick. This is not to say that the pastoral minister's aim is to use the homily to answer all the questions the sick would like to ask about their suffering. The homily should first and foremost help them to see their suffering conditions differently as in the light of the gospel. Seeing their conditions differently may entail raising their hopes for a possible physical cure or healing as well as helping them cope with their suffering conditions even when physical cure or healing is delayed or difficult to achieve. The homily also gives hope of eternal life to those whose illnesses are terminal. The homily should be a source of consolation to God-fearing sufferers.

For the healthy, the homily not only helps them see the sick as important members of the community but also prepares them ahead of time for a possible challenge of faith. A person may be healthy today only to be sick tomorrow.

THE PRESENTATION OF THE HOMILY

In presenting the homily, Lowry also advocates beginning with the *itch* and moving to the *scratch*—from human predicament to the solution born of the gospel.[50] In other words, the pastoral minister should start the delivery of the homily by first telling the story of the sick (the *itch*) before moving into the gospel message (the *scratch*).

Telling the patient's story acts as a way of engaging the listeners and making known the felt need. On the other hand the central message acts as a solution or response to the problem. The patient's story may not always come as a negative experience. Whatever the patient's story, the preacher, being a theological reflector, should be able to use the gospel message and respond to the patient's experiences. This response is for the benefit of the sick and for the whole worshiping community.

We have seen the resourcefulness of using bedside encounter with patients. Listening to patients' stories helps to engage the pastoral minister in theological reflection. When a theological reflection originating from the story of the sick is shared in a homily with the worshiping community in a liturgical celebration, the homily may act as a source of grace to the entire community as well as helping the sick to see their stories as part of the larger divine story.

NOTES

1. William Nichols, *Storytelling the Gospel* (St. Louis, Missouri: Chalice Press, 1999), 2.
2. Ronald J. Allen, *Interpreting the Gospel: An Introduction to Preaching* (St. Louis, Missouri: Chalice Press, 1998), 207.
3. Nichols, 5.
4. Allen, *Interpreting the Gospel,* 208.
5. Ibid., 208.
6. Nichols, *Storytelling the Gospel,* 3.
7. Allen, 29.
8. Power, "Let the Sick Man Call," *The Heythrop Journal* 19 (1978): 256.
9. Joye Gros, *Theological Reflection, Connecting Faith and Life* (Chicago, Illinois: Loyola Press, 2001), 5.
10. Patricia O' Connell Killen and John De Beer, *The Art of Theological Reflection* (New York: Crossroad, 1994), 19.
11. Ibid.
12. Ibid., 21.
13. Robert L. Kinast, *What Are They Saying about Theological Reflection*? (New York: Paulist Press, 2000), 66.
14. Edward O. de Bary, *Theological Reflection: The Creation of Spiritual Power in the Informative Age* (Collegeville, MN.: Liturgical Press, 2003), 42.
15. David A. Hogue, *Remembering the Future Imaging the Past: Story, Ritual, and Human Brain* (Cleveland: The Pilgrim Press, 2003), 100.
16. Carrie Doehring, *The Practice of Pastoral Care: A Post-Modern Approach* (Louisville, KY.: Westminster John Knox Press, 2006), 18.
17. Ibid., 96.
18. Gerard Egan, *Face to Face: The Small-Group Experience and Interpersonal Growth* (Pacific Grove, CA.: Brooks/Cole Publishing Company, 1973), 87.
19. Wayne E. Oates, *The Revelation of God in Human Suffering* (Philadelphia, PA.: The Westminster Press, 1952), 36.
20. Joyce Travelbee, *Interpersonal Aspects of Nursing* (Philadelphia, PA.: F.A. Davis Company, 1971), 66.
21. Ibid.
22. Ibid., 71.

23. Ibid., 70.
24. William Skudlarek, *The Word in Worship: Preaching in a Liturgical Context* (Nashville, TN.: Abingdon, 1981), 11.
25. Ibid., 14.
26. Ibid., 13.
27. Ibid., 15.
28. Allen, 113.
29. Skudlarek, *The Word in Worship*, 31.
30. Ibid., 34.
31. Ibid., 45.
32. Daniel E. Harris, *We Speak the Word of the Lord: A Practical Plan for More Effective Preaching* (Chicago, IL.: ACTA Publications, 2001), 14.
33. Skudlarek., 51.
34. Scott Kevin Davis, *"A Pastoral Care Hermeneutic for Preaching: From Patient Bedside Narrative to Congregational Pulpit Proclamation,"* (Doctor of Ministry in Preaching Thesis, Aquinas Institute of Theology, 2003), 67.
35. Leonora Tubbs Tisdale, *Preaching as Local Theology and Folk Art* (Minneapolis: Fortress Press, 1997), 55.
36. Allen, 66.
37. Eugene L. Lowry, *The Homiletical Plot: The Sermon as Narrative Art Form* (Louisville, Kentucky: Westminster John Knox Press, 2001), 18.
38. E. F. Malone, "Kerygma," in *New Catholic Encyclopedia*, 2002 ed.
39. Lowry, 18.
40. Ibid.
41. Ibid., 19.
42. Ibid.
43. Herbert Anderson and Edward Foley, *Mighty Stories, Dangerous Rituals* (San Franscisco: Jossey-Bass Publishers, 1998), 34.
44. Anderson and Foley, 37.
45. Ibid.
46. Lowry, 19.
47. Ibid., 18.
48. Ibid., 17.
49. Ibid., 19.
50. Ibid., 20.

Chapter Five

The Preaching Evaluation

In this chapter, we shall test the effectiveness of sermons preached with patients' stories as compared to those sermons without patients' stories. The first three homilies were preached with patients' stories while the last three were preached without making any direct reference to the sick and to their experiences. Sermons preached without patients' stories refer to those sermons which focus on the biblical text rather than stories and experiences of patients. The effectiveness of the homilies was tested with a questionnaire designed for hospital patients. Copies of the questionnaires were distributed to patients in their rooms ahead of six Sunday liturgical celebrations and collected after the six liturgies.

Another way these homilies were tested was to engage in face to face conversation with hospital patients, especially those who may not be able to express their feelings in writing by filling in the options as provided in the questionnaire. The health conditions of many patients may make it more difficult for them to write while lying in beds. This face to face conversation with patients is another way of providing a better opportunity for those patients who may find it easier to give more detailed information verbally about the homilies, especially where the questionnaire does not give them enough opportunity. The following two pages include a copy of the questionnaire that was distributed to hospital patients before the six celebrations of Sunday liturgy. These questionnaires were collected later after the Sunday liturgies and used in the evaluation of the effectiveness of applying patients' stories and their experiences in preaching.

A QUESTIONNAIRE FOR THE RESPONSES OF HOSPITAL PATIENTS

After listening to the homily over the television or inside the chapel, check one of these options as the homily appeals to you. You do not need to write your name.

1. How effective was this homily?
   (a) Very effective
   (b) Effective
   (c) Somewhat effective
   (d) Not very effective
2. How well did the homily today address the *feelings* you are encountering right now in your illness?
   (a) Excellent
   (b) Good
   (c) Fair
   (d) Did not help much
3. How well did the homily address the *questions* you are asking right now in your illness?
   (a) Excellent
   (b) Good
   (c) Fair
   (d) Did not help much
4. How well did the homily challenge you to new understanding or insight regarding your illness or suffering in general?
   (a) Excellent
   (b) Good
   (c) Fair
   (d) Did not help much
5. How well did the homily proclaim the goodness and faithfulness of God today even in the midst of illness?
   (a) Excellent
   (b) Good
   (c) Fair
   (d) Did not help much

6a. How important was the patient's story in the effectiveness of this homily for you?
   (a) Very important
   (b) Important

(c) Somewhat important
(d) Not very important
6b. In a few lines, explain a bit further your answer to question 6a? This is optional.
7. Do you have any other comments about the homily? This is also optional.

EVALUATION OF THE QUESTIONNAIRE

In the questionnaire, questions one through five were used to test the effectiveness of both the homilies preached with patients' stories and those preached without patients' stories. Questions 6a through 7 were used to test the homilies preached with patients' stories only.

Questions 1-6a were evaluated by using numerical values, while questions 6b and 7 were evaluated qualitatively by the quality or strength of the comments made by patients. Answers (a) and (b) of the questionnaire were considered as positive reactions. On the other hand, answers (c) and (d) were considered more negatively.

THE RESULTS OF THE QUESTIONNAIRE

The results of the questionnaires are demonstrated in the charts. Chart A shows the results of the homilies preached with patients' stories, while chart B shows the results of the homilies preached without patients' stories.

The results of this questionnaire clearly indicate that most patients prefer homilies preached with their stories and experiences than homilies preached without a reference to what is happening to them. For example in question 1 of Chart A (homilies 1-3), 20 out of 22 patients indicated that the homilies were "Very effective" or "Effective." Only two indicated that the homilies were "Not very effective or Somewhat effective."

EVALUATION OF THE HOMILIES

Charts A demonstrates that a large majority of the patients indicated that the homilies preached with their stories were "Very Effective or Effective." The homilies also addressed the feelings of patients and the questions they were asking about illness. Applying their stories and experiences to homilies challenged them to new understanding about illness and proclaimed the goodness of God even in the midst of illness. In question 6a, all patients responded that

Chart A. Homilies with Patients' Stories

Questions	*Homilies*	*No of Responses*	*Positive*	*Negative*	*Average*
Question 1	Homily 1	8 out of 10	8	0	4
Question 1	Homily 2	7 out of 10	6	1	3.5
Question 1	Homily 3	7 out of 10	6	1	3.5
Question 2	Homily 1	8 out of 10	7	1	4
Question 2	Homily 2	6 out of 10	6	0	3
Question 2	Homily 3	7 out of 10	7	0	3.5
Question 3	Homily 1	8 out of 10	8	0	4
Question 3	Homily 2	6 out of 10	5	1	3
Question 3	Homily 3	6 out of 10	6	0	3
Question 4	Homily 1	8 out of 10	8	0	4
Question 4	Homily 2	6 out of 10	4	2	3
Question 4	Homily 3	7 out of 10	6	1	3.5
Question 5	Homily 1	7 out of 10	7	0	3.5
Question 5	Homily 2	8 out of 10	7	1	4
Question 5	Homily 3	7 out of 10	6	1	3.5
Question 6a	Homily 1	8 out of 10	8	0	4
Question 6a	Homily 2	6 out of 10	6	0	3
Question 6a	Homily 3	7 out of 10	7	0	3.5

the stories of other patients used in the homilies were "Very important" or "Important" in the effectiveness of the homilies.

Only one patient responded to question 6b, an optional choice. According to the respondent, "The patient's story shows a man suffering much more than me. His faith brings me hope." The same single patient responded to

Chart B. Homilies without Patients' Stories

Questions	*Homilies*	*No of Responses*	*Positive*	*Negative*	*Average*
Question 1	Homily 4	7 out of 10	6	1	3.5
Question 1	Homily 5	7 out of 10	6	1	3.5
Question 1	Homily 6	6 out of 10	5	1	3
Question 2	Homily 4	7 out of 10	3	4	3.5
Question 2	Homily 5	7 out of 10	2	5	3.5
Question 2	Homily 6	6 out of 10	2	4	3
Question 3	Homily 4	7 out of 10	2	5	3.5
Question 3	Homily 5	6 out of 10	2	4	3
Question 3	Homily 6	6 out of 10	1	5	3
Question 4	Homily 4	7 out of 10	3	4	3.5
Question 4	Homily 5	7 out of 10	1	6	3.5
Question 4	Homily 6	6 out of 10	1	5	3
Question 5	Homily 4	7 out of 10	5	2	3.5
Question 5	Homily 5	7 out of 10	3	4	3.5
Question 5	Homily 6	5 out of 10	1	4	2.4

question 7: "Thank you for mentioning other forms of suffering, like losing a job." With this single qualitative response, the results of the optional questions are not statistically significant.

Chart B demonstrates the impression of patients about those three homilies preached without patients' stories and experiences. They responded positively but indicated that the homilies did not address their feelings nor the questions they were asking about illness. Nor did these homilies challenge them to new understanding about illness and the goodness of God in the midst of illness.

ANECDOTAL RESPONSES

Apart from the written responses, some patients made more convincing verbal reactions to the homilies when I went to collect the questionnaires in their rooms. One of the patients told me that starting the homily with a patient's story captured his attention and kept him focused on the television till the end of the Mass. The questions which the patient in the story was asking God were also the questions bothering him before the homily. The patient also expressed that his understanding of God's love and place in human suffering became stronger.

Another patient told me that she felt very uncomfortable and frustrated as she did not experience enough relief for the past two days she was in the hospital. She said, "The homily strengthened my endurance and gave me more strength to fight the pains in connection with my knee replacement."

A third patient remarked that she felt frustrated with the difficult nature of her cancer. She was full of denial about what might happen at the end. She was encouraged by the cancer patient in the second homily. She said, "The way the cancer patient handled her painful condition has helped me more to accept and see my illness differently."

Some patients also reacted verbally to the homilies preached without patients' stories. Though they appreciated the homilies as good, they felt that they were better preached to a parish audience and not very suitable for a hospital audience.

THE LIMITATIONS OF THE QUESTIONNAIRE

The questions seemed to have given more of quantitative information, but not much qualitative or in-depth explanation. The last two questions requiring more detailed information were optional. However, due to the health conditions of many of the patients and their inability to give detailed answers in writing, face-to-face conversations about the homilies were provided.

Some of the patients were not able to focus their attention on the homilies because of the distractions that came from hospital workers and visitors. One of the patients complained and said, "Just as I wanted to listen to the homily, my doctor came in to see me. I am sorry, I could not respond to the questions because I did not want to tell lies." Some patients were too weak or in terrible pain and unable to concentrate on the message of the homilies and so did not respond to the questions.

The homilies were plotted with the consciousness that both patients and those who serve them have limited time for liturgical celebrations. Therefore, the homilies were prepared for delivery within seven to ten minutes. The time factor made it difficult to provide more detailed messages as would be suitable for normal church worship. Also, the homilies with patients' stories were designed to concentrate on addressing the problems of the sick. These homilies did not present much about the problems of the healthy members of the hospital community.

Preaching to a hospital community is not the same as preaching to a parish audience. Most of the patients were not able to come into the chapel to take part in the liturgical celebrations and so listened via television. Some of them complained of hearing problems due to the malfunction of their television sets or their noisy surroundings.

Despite all of these limitations, the evaluation process still yielded positive results. These positive results were based on the numerical values of the written responses, and the quality of the anecdotal comments made by patients. The entire responses clearly indicated the importance of including patients' stories and experiences in hospital preaching.

Homilies

Six homilies are presented here. The first three were preached with the stories and experiences of hospitalized patients. The last three were preached without mentioning their stories and experiences. The last three homilies sound like homilies preached to a congregation made up of mostly the healthy members of a community.

HOMILIES WITH PATIENTS' STORIES AND EXPERIENCES

Homily 1. Homily of the 5th Sunday in Ordinary Time in Year B

Texts
1st Reading: Job 7: 1-4, 6-7
2nd Reading: 1 Cor. 9:16, 22-23
3rd Reading: Mk 1:29-39

I was once asked to go and see a young man in his mid thirties who had indicated to his nurse that he had suffered enough and wanted to end his life. Due to a shooting event that took place when he was twenty-five years old, Ken (not his real name) had been paralyzed from waist down for ten years. He was fed up with life after so long in a wheelchair. Ken's doctor had just told him that there was no possibility of his walking again. This sad news was so devastating to him that Ken wished he were dead.

Ken even expressed his disappointment with God for not protecting him in the shooting. After years of prayers, instead of experiencing healing from God, Ken heard the worst news. When I got to the door of his room, I saw a broken man, sad and depressed. I felt sad like him and imagined myself in his condition. I tried my best to give him enough support and concern to help him change the way he saw his condition. Fortunately, he abandoned his earlier plan to take his life. Though he had changed his mind, his story still reminded me of the suffering of many people, like those we heard about today in the readings.

Job felt abandoned by God and overwhelmed by suffering. Job talked like someone who was not only tired of life but also as someone who had a very negative impression about life on earth. He could not understand why he should suffer. However, the problem of suffering did not start or end with Job. Like Ken and others, there are many people in this hospital and outside this hospital who are at this moment feeling the same as Job.

Sometimes, it looks as if life is filled with endless misery and pain. In such troubling conditions, it is not a sin to ask God questions.[1] Are there any satisfactory human explanations for suffering? Truly, there are not. Does God really abandon us in our suffering? Sometimes, difficult circumstances can make us feel forgotten by God as Jesus felt during his Passion. But in a real sense, our faith tells us that God does not abandon us. The feeling of abandonment may indicate the depth of human suffering. Even though it is possible to feel abandoned, it is still our belief that Jesus had so much love for the sick.[2]

In the Gospel of today, Jesus responds practically to human illness and suffering. His response reveals the true image of God and God's compassion to those who are suffering either from illness or from other sources of pain. Jesus was surrounded by a multitude of physically and mentally sick people who needed help. He did not start answering the question of why people suffer. He did not treat them as those who were responsible for their illnesses and so were being punishment by God.

Jesus healed Peter's mother in-law and many other sick people brought to him. He cast out the demons that held them hostage. Jesus showed much concern to the sick in the Gospels, sometimes even contrary to what the culture permitted, to express his support and love for the sick and suffering. He allowed the sick, who in that culture were regarded as sinners, to touch him in order to be healed and be forgiven (Mk. 6: 56, Lk. 8: 43-48,). Jesus touched even the untouchables and healed them (Lk. 5: 13). Jesus listened to the sick and to their concerns (Lk. 7: 2-10). He not only cured and healed the sick but also reconciled them with their communities (Lk. 5:14). He visited the sick in their homes, brought them back to life, and spent time with them (Mk. 5: 21-24). He devoted himself to them and did not even immune himself to their suffering.[3] Jesus also embraced a life of suffering to identify with those who were suffering.

All these activities of Jesus among the sick are clear indications that God does not abandon us in times of hardship and pain. It is not God's plan that we suffer. Hardship and pain continue to be realities of life that we cannot avoid.[4] In obedience to his father's plan, Jesus himself had to accept suffering. The passion of Jesus can be a consolation to all who have faith and who are suffering. The suffering of a Christian could be seen as an opportunity to show one's faith and to share in Christ's suffering with the hope that suffering will not end in Calvary but in the glory of resurrection.[5]

For those of us who work in health facilities, our services among the sick should be seen as an opportunity to take part in spreading the love Jesus has for the suffering. When we do our jobs very well, we provide an opportunity for people to feel the love and care of God. As Peter's mother-in-law waited on Jesus after her healing, some people who receive care from us glorify God and show hospitality to others. It is possible when we treat the sick well with love and care we may feel happy and rewarded.

Homily 2. Homily for the Sixth Sunday in Ordinary Time in Year B

Texts
1st Reading: Lev. 13:-2, 44-46
2nd Reading: 1Cor. 10: 31-11:1
Gospel: Mk. 1:40-45

I once had an encounter with a fifty-year-old cancer patient who surprised me. Jane (not her real name) was in terrible pain. It was not clear if she was going to survive her current hospitalization. Jane was honest and told me how terrible she felt and how much she had suffered. I have seen patients in her condition look very angry and sometimes blame God for what is happening to them. I remember having asked her to tell me how in her condition, she felt about God. Expecting Jane to lash out and blame God for her illness, I was surprised with her response. She said, "If not for God, my illness could have been worse. I have handed myself and this cancer over to God and I am ready for whatever comes." Jane's response was an amazing expression of faith. Jane had accepted a condition she couldn't change and had surrendered herself to whatever God allows or wishes.

In today's gospel, we see a person who had an illness as traumatic as cancer. The leper's expression of faith, acceptance, and submission to the wish of Jesus was remarkable and so surprised Jesus. Leprosy was a most dreaded disease in New Testament times. The leper suffered not only from physical pain but also from mental torture and social isolation. Walking along the road, the leper would have to ring the bell shouting "unclean" and people would run away from him. Parents, relations, and friends disowned such a person. A leper was asked to live alone outside the community. The leper was alive, but dead. People believed the leper was unclean and cursed by God. It was in this hopeless and desperate situation that the leper in today's gospel met Jesus.

The leper said to Jesus, "If you wish, you can make me clean." One would have expected the leper to rush to beg Jesus to grant his wish to be healed. Though he wished to be healed, he was still ready to accept whatever was the wish of Jesus. In other words, if healing came as fast as he wanted, he would glorify God. If healing did not come the way he wanted, he was still ready to accept what he could not change while still hoping for God's intervention and mercy. He had no doubt that Jesus had the powers to help him. However, considering the seriousness of the disease and the taboo surrounding it, the leper made a bold move.

The reaction of Jesus to this man's illness shows the love Jesus has for the sick. Jesus did not treat the leper as one who was responsible for his illness. Jesus did not mind the onlookers, who regarded a leper as an unapproachable. Jesus took pity on the leper and stretched out his hands and touched him. This action of touching a leper was a shocking behavior and not expected of any serious religious person. However, Jesus' action was not only a symbolic act of love but also a way of teaching us how to care for the sick. It is important to observe all the safety measures when approaching those with infectious diseases. At the same time, we do not need to run away from our sick brothers and sisters.

The response of Jesus to the leper shows that God is ready to helps us recover from our illnesses, irrespective of how serious they are. To be sick may not be a blessing, and no person wishes to be sick. At the same time, it is one of those realities of life we often experience. When one is sick, it is natural to hope for healing as fast as possible. It is frustrating when healing does not come as fast as we expect. This does not mean that God has forsaken us. When illness comes, it may be considered a test of our faith and trust in God.

Our faith assures us that God is always with us and even suffers with us. Jesus invites all who are labored and burdened, and he will give them rest. Jesus not only cured the leper of his physical illness but also healed him by reconciling him with his community. Jesus asked him to go and show himself to the priest and offer sacrifice to show the community that he was healed and ready to be accepted back with his family, friends, and relations.

As Jesus cured and healed the leper in today's gospel, we pray that through our services, support, and prayers, God will bring healing to all who are sick.

No matter how difficult the illnesses, God is capable of granting mercy and healing. Like the leper in today's gospel, we may manage our illness better by our hope, patience, and steadfastness in times of trial.

Homily 3. Homily of the 7th Sunday in Ordinary Time Year B

Texts:
1st Reading: Is. 43: 18-19, 21-22, 24b-25
2nd Reading: 2Cor. 1:18-22
3rd Reading: Mk 2:1-12

When I entered her room, I could not make out from her facial expression how she was feeling. Ms. Alphonso (not her real name) was 87 years old, though she looked far younger than her age. I saw a basketful of beautiful flowers at her bedside. I was attracted to their brightness and fragrance. I said, "Ma'am, look at these beautiful flowers. I see beautiful pictures and the names of beautiful children hanging on these colorful flowers. Please tell me about these flowers and the pictures hanging on them."

Her response was immediate. She beamed a smile and spoke, "Father, I'm so blessed. My son has just come from California with two of my grandkids to visit me. They brought these flowers. The little pictures on the flowers are of my grand and great-grand children. I have twenty grand-children and five great-grand children. Many of my children live in different parts of the country. My children call me everyday and some in St. Louis visit me everyday." Ms. Alphonso further told me how God had blessed her with very caring and loving family members, relations, and friends.

Though her illness kept her a bit uncomfortable, she told me that she felt much better, especially when her loved ones were all around her. Despite her illness, I saw her as a happy woman. At least, she was not a lonely woman. Ms. Alphonso's story made me feel that many sick people are happy and find it easier to cope with their illnesses, not simply because they are recovering quickly, but also because of the love, support and care they receive from their families and friends.

In the gospel of today, we saw a beautiful example of how the efforts and the faith of relations, brothers and sisters, and friends can facilitate healing and physical cure. A paralyzed man was brought to Jesus by four men, possibly his relations or brothers. When they could not get to Jesus because of the crowd, they climbed on top of the roof of the house, made an opening on the roof, and lowered the man down to Jesus. Imagine and reflect a little, as if you are looking at four men lifting a sick man on top of a roof. See how they work as a team for the healing of their sick brother. It is an amazing show of love and faith. Their faith was able to break through the obstacle of the crowd. Faith can overcome all obstacles.[6]

This effort and show of faith was not wasted. Jesus was impressed by their faith and responded by healing the man and also forgiving all his sins. The action of Jesus shows that he has the power to heal both the illness of the body and that of the soul. By first forgiving the man's sin, Jesus implied that sin is an illness of the soul. Jesus did not distinguish between the sickness of the body and the sickness of the soul.[7] Jesus took care of the paralytic man's body and soul because bodily illness can also be connected to the illness of the soul. Just as we care for the physical wellbeing of one another, we should also care for their spiritual wellbeing. Without the efforts of his friends, the paralyzed man would not have had access to the healing mercy of Jesus.

The four friends of the paralyzed man, however, were not responsible for his healing but their response to his needs brought about Christ's healing and forgiveness of sin.[8] Their action truly reduced or put a stop to the suffering of their friend. Many people have received healing because of the medical care they received, as well as of the support of their loved ones. From my own experiences, having worked in a hospital for many years, the happiest patients are those who have the full support of their families and friends. Even those whose illnesses are terminal die happily when family members, friends, and relations surround them during their final moments.

Let us therefore continue giving our support to our loved ones who are ill. Our support is as needed as the other services they receive in the hospital. When we are with them, they feel less abandoned and healing may come faster.

HOMILIES WITHOUT REFERENCE TO STORIES AND EXPERIENCES OF THE SICK

Homily 4. Homily for the First Week of Lent: Year B

Texts
1st Reading: Gen. 9: 8-15
2nd Reading: 1 Pet. 3:18-22
3rd Reading: Mk. 1:12-15.

When I was a young man in Nigeria, I was required to join the National Youth Service Corp (NYSC), a para-military group. NYSC exposed young adults to military experiences in order to be prepared to serve their country. During the training, I was in camp and remember what happened when one of our military instructors was teaching us how to protect ourselves from enemy fire. Some of us who did not see ourselves as aspiring professional soldiers were not serious about the instructions.

Consequently, the military officer said, "You'd better take what I am telling you seriously because these skills are important. I am talking from experience. You may not want to be professional soldiers. Still, anyone of you could be attacked any time and so you need these skills. If I had not experienced the dangers of battlefield, I wouldn't be telling you this." His statement, that he was talking from experience and that anyone could be attacked, made a lot of sense to me. It is always better for someone who has undergone an experience to give others instructions.

In the gospel of today, Jesus experienced the temptation of the devil like any of us, but did not sin. How could the Son of God be tempted by the devil? If the Son of God was not free from the temptation of the devil, who is then free? His temptation, of course, was part of his solidarity with us, in order to teach us from his own experience. It is always better and more convincing for one who has undergone an experience to teach others. It is more convincing for someone who has survived suffering or hardship to pass on to others how to endure. By taking flesh, the Son of God subjected himself to all human conditions. It is not surprising that he was not immune to suffering, to hurt, to disappointment, and to temptation.[9] He couldn't have taught us better how to fight and defeat the devil if he had not fought and defeated the devil himself.

How did Jesus defeat the devil? Though the gospel of Mark did not narrate in detail how Jesus prepared himself in the wilderness to face the devil, Matthew and Luke give a better account of what happened. Jesus subjected himself to some spiritual discipline. He went into the desert and spent forty days and forty nights fasting and praying. He was also knowledgeable with the sacred writings. The Son of God did not take the devil for granted. Why would any of us not prepare for possible temptations that could come at any moment in our lives? No wonder the Church encourages us during the Lenten period to share in the experiences of our Master.

This season of Lent offers us the opportunity to subject ourselves to some religious practices that can help us to be spiritually strong. We are encouraged to spend more time in prayer. Prayer helps us to fight temptations. Prayer is like a bullet-proof vest or helmet which a soldier wears in battle to be protected from enemy fire. No wonder Jesus asked his sleepy disciples at the Garden of Gethsemane to watch and to pray.

We are also encouraged to abstain from some pleasures in order to control our desires. Jesus was able to withstand the temptation of satisfying his hunger and of showing his power because he learned how to survive without them. We need to engage in some acts of generosity to help our brothers and sisters in need. God has been very generous to us and so we should be ready to share what God has given to us with others who are not as privileged as we are. Through generosity, we can also receive grace and forgiveness of sin. The Church understands that in this life it is difficult if not impossible to avoid being tempted.[10] As this is the first week of Lent, we have enough time to be serious with these religious practices in order to boost our spiritual strength.

Homily 5. Homily for Easter Sunday Year B

Texts
1st Reading: Acts 10:34.37-43
2nd Reading: Col. 3:1-4
3rd Reading: Jn. 20:1-9

Last April, at around 3:00 a.m. in the morning, my phone rang continuously. Initially I did not want to pick up the call because it was unusual for me to get calls at that time of the night. When the phone kept ringing, I decided to pick up. I was shocked at the news that my immediate younger brother had died. I was crushed and heartbroken. I found it hard to believe because this was the first time I had ever experienced the death of a young and close blood relation. It seemed like a dream but still seemed true. I could not sleep again, wondering what might have caused his death. I had prayed and wished for another phone call telling me that the doctors had applied some last measures and had revived him. I imagined how happy I would feel if I got another phone call declaring him not dead, but alive again.

Though my wish to hear that he was alive did not come true, this experience helped me to imagine and understand how happy the disciples of Christ felt on hearing that he was alive again. Jesus' followers, who had witnessed their master's Passion and cruel execution on the cross, heard the best news of their lives—Jesus had risen from the dead. It was not a dream but a reality. Mary Magdalene had gone to the tomb on the first day of the week, but found it empty. There was initial skepticism and confusion about whether the empty tomb really meant that Jesus was alive or that his body had been stolen. Peter and John ran down to the tomb to confirm what the woman had told them. They were no longer confused when Jesus appeared to them and showed them his arms and legs. Jesus not only appeared to them, but also ate and drank with them, thereby establishing the continuity between his early life and his glorified life.[11] Rising from the dead, however, does not mean returning to the same earthly life he used to live, but rather rising to a glorified life, which death can no longer touch.[12]

The resurrection of Christ meant a lot to his disciples. Before their master rose from the dead, they had been crushed, disappointed, afraid, and disorganized. For them, the resurrection meant a transformation to a new life. Their fears and disappointments were over and Easter was a time for them to bear witness with courage and boldness. As we saw in the first reading, Peter fearlessly addressed the same people he had been afraid of and who had crucified his master. Without fear, Peter asked the congregation to believe in Jesus and receive forgiveness.

My brothers and sisters, by gathering today to take part in this celebration, we are sharing in the joys, blessings, and challenges of Easter. The resurrection should also mean a lot to us. It should also mean a rising to a new life. It is a celebration that gives meaning to our faith and hope to our lives. For those who believe, the resurrection of Christ assures us that there is hope that after death, we have a glorified life to live in eternity.

The discipline of Lent was an opportunity for us to get rid of our old, sinful ways and receive God's forgiveness in order to gain from the transforming effect of Easter. To benefit from the blessings of this glorious celebration, we are called to bear witness by a new way of living our lives in obedience to God's commandment of loving God and one another.

Homily 6. Homily for the Fifth Sunday of Easter Year B

Texts
1st Reading: Acts 9:26-31
2nd Reading: 1 Jn. 3:18-24
3rd Reading: Jn. 15:1-8

Today is the day we celebrate and honor our mothers as special blessings from God. Mothers have sacrificed greatly to nurture, provide, guide, and protect us in life. In good times and in bad times, mothers have always been our strength and support. Today's celebration is an opportunity for us to pray for our mothers and to express our love and gratitude to them. Without the love, the care, and the nurturing of our mothers, it would have been very difficult for us to survive and to be what we are today. We owe them a lot.

Though the readings of today do not have direct reference to the Mother's Day celebration, still, the close relationship that should exist between a mother and child helps us to understand the imagery Jesus used to describe the relationship that should exist between him and his disciples. Jesus said to his disciples, "I am the vine, you are the branches." By this statement, Jesus describes the closeness, unity, and interdependence that should exist between him and his disciples. Jesus wants us to understand who he is and who we are.[13] He is our master and we are his members. As St Paul puts it, we are "the members of the body of Christ."

We are therefore invited as individuals and as communities to have a relationship with Jesus. How blessed and privileged are we to have a relationship with Jesus? We must not miss this divine opportunity. To grasp the importance of this relationship and to be part of it, we must understand the type of attachment, dependence, and interdependence that should exist between the vine and the branches. The branch must remain attached to the vine in order to remain alive. The vine extracts mineral resources from the soil, exposes them to the sun, and feeds the branches. To bear fruit, the branches need to remain attached to the vine. Nothing good comes from branches if they remain apart from the vine. When a branch is cut off from the vine, it dies and withers away.

In like manner, or just as the branches need the vine, we need Christ. He is the source of life and everything good in us. Severed from him, there is no life in us and we cannot bear fruit. We must therefore keep close contact with Christ. How do we keep close contact with Christ? We must be constant in our prayers. We must learn how our Master kept close contact with his Father. "The secret of the life of Jesus was his contact with God; again and again he withdrew into a solitary place to meet him."[14] Jesus had the habit of consulting his Father in prayer before making any major decisions. Before he started his public ministry, Jesus went into the wilderness and prayed for forty days and forty nights. Before he chose his disciples, he went to a secret place to pray. Before his Passion, he went to the mountain top with three disciples to have contact with his Father and his messengers. Prayer is always our major contact with God.

Another way we can keep in contact with Christ is to allow ourselves to be pruned by the Word of God. The Word of God makes known to us the perfect words and actions of our Master. We must, therefore, model our daily lives according to the ways of Christ. Since Christian life and fruitfulness come from the vine only, Jesus is the only source of our goodness. Jesus lived a selfless life of service to make others feel the love and presence of God. By so doing, he taught us how to care for one another.

As the vine needs the branches, Jesus also needs us. Jesus needs us to bear good fruit in our communities and in the world at large. How do we do it? "Each of us has some gift. By developing, using, and sharing that gift with others, we become fruitful."[15] Many of us here are talented doctors, pharmacists, nurses, social workers, therapists, or chaplains. Being fruitful is being able to use our gifts to serve others, especially the sick. Our fruitfulness or services should help people experience the love, care, and the presence of God.

The best way to prove that we are true disciples of Christ is to bear good fruit in our actions and in our words. When we bear good fruit we recognize the dignity and value of each person. We attend to the needs of others as best as we can and we help one another to be all that we can be in our community of faith. At times, this can bring healing, and sometimes, this can bring happiness. Our actions and words should always bring care and comfort and these should reflect God's nearness.

NOTES

1. William Nichols, *Storytelling the Gospel* (St. Louis, Missouri: Chalice Press, 1999), 3.
2. Stephen F. Brett, "Preparing for the Finals," *Homiletic and Pastoral Review*, (January 2009): 35-37.
3. Ibid.
4. Noel Quesson, *Pray with the Bible: Fifth Sunday of the Year*, Vol. VII (Bangalore, India: Theological Publication, 1994), 162.
5. Flor McCarthy, *New Sunday and Holy Day Liturgies, New Sunday and Holy Day Liturgies: Year B* (Dublin, Ireland: Dominican Publication, 1998), 184.
6. Noel Quesson, *Pray with the Bible: Fifth Sunday of the Year*, Vol. VII (Bangalore, India: Theological Publication, 1994), 174.
7. Flor McCarthy, *New Sunday and Holy Day Liturgies: Year B* (Dublin, Ireland: Dominican Publication, 1998), 194.
8. Stephen F. Brett, "Preparing for the Finals," *Homiletic and Pastoral Review*, (January 2009): 39-40.
9. Flor McCarthy, *New Sunday and Holy Day Liturgies: Year B* (Dublin, Ireland: Dominican Publication, 1998), 67.
10. William Barclay, *The Daily Study Bible: The Gospel of Mark* (Bangalore, India: Theological Publications in India, 1999), 21.
11. Timothy J. Cronin, "Homily Helps: Easter Sunday," *St Anthony's Messenger*, 12 April 2009, 1.
12. Flor McCarthy, *New Sunday and Holy Day Liturgies: Year B* (Dublin, Ireland: Dominican Publication, 1998), 102.
13. Noel Quesson, *Pray with the Bible: Fifth Sunday of the Year*, Vol. VII (Bangalore, India: Theological Publication, 1994), 120.
14. William Barclay, *The Daily Study Bible: The Gospel of John* (Bangalore, India: Theological Publications in India, 1999), 176.
15. Flor McCarthy, *New Sunday and Holy Day Liturgies: Year B* (Ireland, Dublin: Dominican Publication, 1998), 126.

Conclusion

My motivation for carrying out this research was to discover more about my pastoral observation that more intentional hospital bedside listening to the stories and experiences of the sick is very necessary for effective hospital preaching to the sick. I was also wondering whether the use of patients' stories and experiences in homilies had any influence on the effectiveness of my preaching to the hospital community made up of the sick, their relations, friends, and the hospital staff.

The effective use of patients' stories and experiences in preaching requires offering them "hospitality," that is a free and friendly space to express themselves to be listened to. A review of what some experts have experienced about offering hospitality to the sick helped me to learn about valuable information that can be used in preaching. I also learned that listening to the sick express their feelings about their illnesses offers an opportunity for the pastoral minister to help them find meaning in their suffering. This meaning can facilitate healing or, at least, may help the sick cope with illness.

The importance of hospitality to the sick became more evident to me when I visited a young man who had planned to take his own life after a shooting incident that paralyzed him. My encounter with this patient helped him to see his condition differently. As a result of our conversation, he changed his mind and decided to move on with life. I used his story in one of my homilies. The positive feedback I got from other patients who listened to the homily encouraged me to keep using patients' stories and experiences in preaching.

Hospitality to the sick is not only helpful to them but also to the pastoral minister and to the community. By listening to the sick narrate their stories and experiences, the pastoral minister and the community realize the importance of the sick and what the sick can offer to the community. When their stories are shared in a liturgical context, the sick can become a sacrament or a source of grace to the healthy members of the community. My bedside encounters with patients and their relations after Sunday liturgies also made me know the importance of sharing patients' stories in liturgical celebrations. Some family members expressed how the homilies had helped them to understand better God's role in the healing process of their loved ones. Some health workers who took part in the liturgies also confessed better understanding of their roles in the healing process of their patients. After listening to the third homily, one of the nurses said, "I now see myself more as an instrument God is using to effect healing."

Encountering the sick involves meaningful interpersonal communication. For this communication to be effective, the pastoral minister needs to use strong communication skills. It is the responsibility of the pastoral minister to learn and practice good conversational skills so as to build pastoral relationships. When there is good rapport, the patient communicates more openly. In my routine room-to-room visitation of the sick, I applied some rapport skills as I listened and conversed. They expressed themselves freely and related their private stories and experiences. Their cooperation with me shows the extent a pastoral minister needs good conversational skills to be able to minister effectively.

The use of patients' stories and experiences in preaching involves theological reflection which the pastoral minister initiates. A theological reflector begins reflecting on the experiences of the patient to find new meaning in accordance with the religious tradition of the patient. After reflecting theologically on these stories, the pastoral minister may also share these stories with the community in liturgical celebrations.

The movement of patients' stories from bedside to pulpit involves a three-way hermeneutical process. This three-way hermeneutical process includes an interpretation of the patient's community, the patient's story, and God's own story (Biblical text) from the lectionary. The interpretation of patients' stories revealed some problems (fear, pain, abandonment, anger, depression, etc) while the interpretation of the Biblical texts revealed some kerygmatic themes that provided clues for resolutions. The interpretation of the patient's community helped me to address my hospital audience in context.

After carrying out this three-way hermeneutical process, I prepared three homilies using patients' stories as well as the Biblical text. In the preparation of each homily, I ritualized the patient's story by linking God's story and the human story in order to help the patient reconstruct his life and see his story as part of the divine story. I utilized Eugene Lowry's ideas of forming and shaping a sermon by the interaction of problem and theme. These three homilies were delivered using Lowry's ideas of beginning with the *itch* and moving to the *scratch*—from human predicament to the solution born of the gospel. This method involves the delivery of the homily by first telling the story of the sick (the *itch*) before moving into the Gospel message (the *scratch*).

To test the effectiveness of sermons preached with patients' stories as compared to those sermons without patients' stories, I prepared three other homilies with out patients' stories as presented in the appendix. The effectiveness of the homilies was tested with a questionnaire designed to give hospital patients opportunities to express their feelings about the homilies. In addition to gathering information from patients' responses to the questionnaire, I conversed face-to-face with patients.

The evaluations of the six homilies seemed to support my thesis. An overwhelming majority of the patients felt that the homilies preached with their stories addressed them more effectively in their conditions than homilies preached without their stories. Some of the patients who spoke to me during our face-to-face conversations expressed how the homilies with patients' stories had helped them to understand God's role in their situations and so were reinforced to cope and to keep fighting for healing. These positive responses affirm my observation that applying patients' stories and experiences in homilies make preaching to the hospital community more effective.

Bibliography

Acosta, Judith and Judith Simon Prager. *The Worst Is Over: What To Say When Every Moment Counts*. San Diego, California: Jodere Group, 2003.

Allen, Ronald J. *Interpreting the Gospel: An Introduction to Preaching*. St. Louis, Missouri: Chalice Press, 1998.

Anderson, Harlene. *Conversation, Language, and Possibilities: A Postmodern Approach to Therapy*. New York: BasicBooks, 1997.

Anderson, Herbert and Edward Foley. *Mighty Stories, Dangerous Rituals*. San Francisco, California: Jossey-Bass Publishers, 1998.

Axtell, Roger E. *Gestures: The Do's and Taboos of Body Language around the World*. New York: John Wiley and Sons Inc., 1998.

Back, Les. *The Act of Listening*. Oxford, England: Berg, 2007.

Bales, Roberts Freed. *Communication, Language, and Meaning: Communication in Small Groups*. New York: Basic Books, 1973.

Barclay, William. *The Daily Study Bible: The Gospel of Mark*. Bangalore, India: Theological Publications in India, 1999.

Baxter, A. Leslie and Barbara M. Montgomery. *Relating: Dialogues and Dialetics*. New York: The Guilford Press, 1996.

Bergant, Dianne, ed. *The Collegeville Bible Commentary: Old Testament*. Collegeville, Minnesota: 1992.

Boothman, Nicholas. *How To Make People Like You in 90 Seconds or Less*. New York: Workman Publishing, 2000.

———. *How To Make People Love You in 90 Seconds or Less*. New York: Workman Publishing, 2004.

Brett, Stephen F. "Preparing for the Finals." *Homiletic and Pastoral Review*, (January 2009): 39-40.

Brunell, Martha. "Hibiscus Blaze," An unpublished article on pastoral care of ALS Patient, St. Louis, 1.

———. *Dear Bradie, A Story of Life with ALS,* narrated, recorded and produced by Douglas D. Cripe, 2006, CD recording.

Cronin, Timothy J. "Homily Helps: Easter Sunday." *St. Anthony Messenger*, 12 April 2009.

David, Mark. "Homily Helps: 7th Sunday in Ordinary Time." *St. Anthony Messenger*, 22 February 2009.

Davis, Scott Kevin. *A Pastoral Care Hermeneutic for Preaching: From Patient Bedside Narrative to Congregational Pulpit Proclamation.* Doctor of Ministry in Preaching Thesis, Aquinas Institute of Theology, 2003.

De Bary, Edward O. *Theological Reflection: The Creation of Spiritual Power in the Informative Age.* Collegeville, Minnesota: Liturgical Press, 2003.

Doehring, Carrie. *The Practice of Pastoral Care: A Post Modern Approach.* Louisville, Kentucky: Westminster John Knox Press, 2006.

Duff, Kat. *The Alchemy of Illness.* New York: Bell Tower, 1993.

Egan, Gerard. *Face to Face: The Small-Group Experience and Interpersonal Growth.* Pacific Grove, California: Brooks/Cole Publishing Company, 1973.

Frankl, Viktor E. *Man's Search for Meaning.* New York: Pocket Books, 1984.

Gros, Joye. *Theological Reflection: Connecting Faith and Life.* Chicago, Illinois: Loyola Press, 2001.

Hensell, Eugene. "Homily Helps: 5th Sunday in Ordinary Time." *St. Anthony Messenger*, 8 February 2009.

Hogue, David A. *Remembering the Future Imaging the Past: Story, Ritual, and Human Brain.* Cleveland, Ohio: The Pilgrim Press, 2003.

Jorgenson, Jane. "Re-relationalizing Rapport in Interpersonal Settings." In *Social Approaches to Communication,* edited by Wendy Leeds-Hurwitz, New York: Guilford Press, 1979.

Kelly, Eugene W. *Effective Interpersonal Communication: A Manual for Skill Development.* Washington, D.C.: University Press of America, 1979.

Killen, Patricia O' Connell and John De Beer. *The Art of Theological Reflection.* New York: Crossroad, 1994.

Kinast, Robert L. *What Are They Saying about Theological Reflection*? New York: Paulist Press, 2000.

Kobak, David. "Homily Helps: First Sunday of Lent." *St. Anthony Messenger*, 1 March 2009.

Kratz, Dennis M. and Abby Robinson Kratz. *Effective Listening Skills.* Chicago, Illinois: Mirror Press, 1995.

Leathers, Dale G. *Successful Nonverbal Communication: Principles and Applications.* Boston, Massachusetts: Allyn and Bacon, 1997.

Lowndes, Leil. *How To Talk to Anyone: 92 Little Tricks for Big Success in Relationships.* New York: Contemporary Books, 2003.

Lowry, Eugene L. *The Homiletical Plot: The Sermon as Narrative Art Form.* Louisville, Kentucky: Westminster John Knox Press, 2001.

McCarthy, Flor. *New Sunday and Holy Day Liturgies: Year B.* Dublin, Ireland: Dominican Publication, 1998.

Meadow, Charles T. *Making Connections: Communication through the Ages.* New York: Scarecrow Press Inc., 2002.

Mehrabian, Albert. *Nonverbal Communication.* Chicago, Illinois: Aldine, 1972.

Morris, Desmond. *Bodytalk: The Meaning of Human Gestures.* New York: Crown Trade Paperbacks, 1994.
Newhouse, Jan. *Moon Dance: Life through the Cancer Lens.* St. Louis, Missouri: Avery Publishing, 2004.
Nichols, William. *Storytelling the Gospel.* St. Louis, Missouri: Chalice Press, 1999.
Norton, Robert. *Communicator Style: Theory, Application, and Measures.* Beverly Hills, California: Sage Publications, 1983.
Nouwen, Henri. *Reaching Out: The Movements of the Spiritual Life.* New York: Doubleday Publishing Company, 1975.
Oates, Wayne E. *The Revelation of God in Human Suffering.* Philadelphia, Pennsylvania: The Westminster Press, 1952.
Power, David N. "Let the Sick Man Call," *The Heythrop Journal* 19 (1978): 256-270.
Purdy, Michael and Deborah Borisoff. Eds., *Listening in Everyday Life.* New York: University Press of America, 1997.
Quesson, Noel. *Pray with the Bible: Fifth Sunday of the Year*, Vol. VII. Bangalore, India: Theological Publication of India, 1994.
Reeves, Donald. "Homily Helps: 6th Sunday in Ordinary Time." *St. Anthony Messenger*, 15 February 2009.
Richmond, Virginia P. and James C. McCroskey. *Nonverbal Behavior in Interpersonal Relations.* Boston, Massachusetts: Pearson, 2004.
Sanford, John A. *Between People: Communicating One-To-One.* New York: Paulist Press, 1982.
Shorter, John. *Conversational Realities: Constructing Life Through Language.* London: Sage Publications, 1994.
Shudlarek, William. *The Word in Worship: Preaching in a Liturgical Context.* Nashville, Tennessee: Abingdon, 1981.
Stone, Richard. *The Healing Art of Storytelling: A Sacred Journey of Personal Discovery.* New York: Author Choice Press, 2004.
Thomlison, T. Dean. *Toward Interpersonal Dialogue.* New York: Longman, 1982.
Tisdale, Leonora Tubbs. *Preaching as Local Theology and Folk Art.* Minneapolis, MN.: Fortress Press, 1997.
Tracy, Karen. *Everyday Talk: Building and Reflecting Identities.* New York: The Guilford Press, 2002.
Travelbee, Joyce. *Interpersonal Aspects of Nursing.* Philadelphia, Pennsylvania: F.A. Davis Company, 1971.
Vargas, Majorie Fink. *Louder Than Words: An Introduction to Non Verbal Communication.* Ames, Iowa: Iowa State University Press, 1986.
Verbrugge, Verlyn D. *The NIV Topical Study Bible: Hospitality.* Grand Rapids, Michigan: Zondervan Bible Publishers, 1989.
Watson, W. Kittie and Larry L. Barker. *Interpersonal and Relational Communication.* Scottsdale, Arizona: Gorsuch Scarisbrick Publishers, 1990.
Whitehead, James D. and Evelyn Eaton Whitehead. *Methods in Ministry: Theological Reflection and Christian Ministry.* Kansas City, Missouri: Sheed and Ward, 1995.
Wolff, Florence I. and Nadine C. Marsnik, *Perceptive Listening.* New York: Harcourt Brace Jovanovich College Publishers, 1995.

Index

Page references in *italics* indicate a chart or table.

About the Author

Cajetan Ngozika Ihewulezi, CSSP, is a Catholic priest of the Holy Ghost order, from Nigeria. After his priestly ordination in 1991, he served as the Vocation Movement Director of the Holy Ghost fathers and brothers of the Nigerian province from 1991-1995. He became the parish priest of Mater Misericordiae, Port Harcourt from 1996-2001. Ihewulezi later traveled to the United States of America for further studies. He received his first Master's degree at Duquesne University in Systematic Theology and a second master's at St. Louis University in Historical Theology. He received a doctorate at Aquinas Institute of Theology. While doing his theological studies at St Louis, he was also trained as a hospital chaplain. He became a board certified hospital chaplain in 2007. Ihewulezi served as a part time hospital chaplain in St Louis Hospital, Barnes Jewish Hospital, St Anthony's Hospital, Forest Park Hospital, and Missouri Baptist Medical Center. He is the author of *Clearing Doubts on Controversial Catholic Doctrines*, *Beyond the Color of Skin*, *The History of Poverty in a Rich and Blessed America*, *Not Created to Come Last*, *Achieving Your Dreams*, *Forward March to Professionalism,* and *Keep Moving Forward.*

Breinigsville, PA USA
23 November 2010
249879BV00003B/2/P

9 780761 852926